General practice as if people mattered

Collected medical essays 1998-2017

Dr Gervase Vernon

To the patients at John Tasker House
and the clients at "Freedom from torture"
whom I have had the privilege to serve

Table of contents

List of papers

(1) Vernon G. The limitations of natural science as applied to medicine. Br J Gen Pract 2002;52(483):870-1.

(2) Vernon G. Essay - What is man? Br J Gen Pract 2003;53:504-5.

(3) Vernon J. Immunisation policy: from compliance to concordance. Br J Gen Pract 2003;53:399-404.

(4) Vernon G. Can there be a moral dialogue between doctor and patient. Catholic Medical Quarterly 2001 Aug.

(5) Vernon G. Teaching tips: balloons and teddy bears. *Evidence-based Medicine* 2006; 11:39.

(6) Vernon G. In a medical bookshop. Br J Gen Pract 2007 Feb;57(535):161.

(7) Vernon G. As water is to fish, so is society to people. Br J Gen Pract 2011 Jan;61(582):74-5.

(8) Vernon G. Between "thisness and quiddity", the place of the general practitioner. Br J Gen Pract 2013 Jul;63(612):373.

(9) Vernon G, Feldman R. Government proposes to end free health care for "failed asylum seekers". Br J Gen Pract 2006 Jan;56(522):59.

(10) Vernon G. A light bulb moment. Br J Gen Pract. 2016 Jul;66(648):379. doi: 10.3399/bjgp16X68600

(11) Vernon G. An Alarm Bell. Br J Gen Pract. 2008 Apr;58(549):285. doi: 10.3399/bjgp08X280010

(12) Vernon G, Ridley D, Lesetedi D. "Home Office syndrome". Br J Gen Pract. 2008 Jul;58(552):510. doi: 10.3399/bjgp08X319530

(13) Vernon G. How to teach trainees about primary care for refugees and asylum seekers. Education for primary care 2008;19(4):430

(14) Vernon G. Denunciation; a new threat to health care for undocumented migrants. Br J Gen Pract. 2012 Feb;62(595):98-9. doi: 10.3399/bjgp12X625265

(15) Vernon G. Working with Polish migrants. Br J Gen Pract 2015; 65 (632 2015; 65:138-632.

(16) Vernon G. The NHS; have the rivets popped? Br J Gen Pract 2017; 67(660):309.doi:10.3399/bjgp17X691385

(17) Vernon G. The lost sheep. Br J Gen Pract. 2017 Nov;67(664):517 doi: 10.3399/bjgp17X693329

ACKNOWLEDGMENTS

With many thanks to Professor Nicky Britten and the other members of the MSc course at King's College without whom these essays would never have been written. With thanks to the BJGP (British Journal of General Practice), where many of these articles were published, for permission to republish them.

Introduction

For the title; "General Practice as if people mattered" I am indebted, of course, to the economist E. F. Schumacher's book; "Economics as if people mattered." Is this title to a collection of essays, all written while I was a full time general practitioner, just a trick to catch the reader's eye, or does it have a link with the contents? Since I started in General Practice in 1984, GP consultations in the UK have been allotted a ridiculously short ten minutes. Nevertheless, every successive government has tried to muscle in on these precious ten minutes, stealing them, as it were, from the patient and the doctor. Governments seek to fill this time with their own good ideas; preventive health care, cervical smears, QOF[1] and so on. Yet, it seems to me, any spare time in the consultation should be spent on the relationship between the patient and the doctor, as if, indeed, the patient mattered. This focus on the relationship between patient and doctor unites many of these otherwise disparate pieces.

None of these pieces has a clinical content. I spent many years learning clinical medicine, then practising and finally teaching it, all of which I enjoyed[2]. The focus on the non-clinical is rather a reflection of a second stage of my life. When I started in General Practice I thought people came to see me for my shiny doctor's bag; for my up to date knowledge. Gradually the bag lost its sheen. I began to realise that people came to see me, not so much for my

---

[1] QOF, the Quality and Outcomes Framework is a system for the performance management and payment of general practitioners which was introduced in 2004. For a further discussion see page 96.

[2] I wrote two pieces which might be considered textbooks. In Malawi in 1981 I wrote a paediatric ward manual for Likuni hospital in Malawi. This has long been overtaken by the paediatric textbook for Malawi written by Dr John Phillips and his colleagues. In 1985 I contributed to the text for a set of slides on venereal disease in developing countries which were distributed by TALC (Teaching Aids at Low Cost). I sometimes think with a wry smile that that may have been my most widely read work.

doctor's bag, but for a piece of me, for a relationship between themselves and a doctor they could trust.

The first three pieces are essays which set out to make a comprehensive review of the nature of general practice. "The limitations of natural science as applied to science" examines the scientific base of medicine, "What is man", considers the nature of man and society, while "What is a general practitioner" reviews the literature about general practice and brings out some underlying features from which certain consequences follow. I return to these themes in other pieces in this collection; the nature of the human person in the short story "Darwin's dream", the nature of the consultation in "Thisness and quiddity". I make no apology for returning to the same subjects and attacking them from different angles and in different genres, for, to me, external reality can be grasped, but never fully understood, in different and complimentary ways, by science and the arts.

After the three initial connected pieces, there follow three longer pieces. The first is a study on the sociology of immunisations called "Immunisation; from compliance to concordance." Unlike the other essays which were written in the odd hour snatched from a busy practice and the duties of family life, this one was researched over a year on Thursday afternoons spent in Cambridge University library. The next, "Beyond altruism" is the summary of a piece of qualitative research on altruism which formed part of my MSc in general practice. It is fitting here to record my gratitude to Professor Nicky Britten and her colleagues who ran the MSc in General Practice course at King's College, London. Without them these pieces would not have been written. The third is a study in ethics; "Can there be a moral dialogue between doctor and patient." In this piece I argue that a doctor, who believes abortion is wrong, can counsel a woman seeking an abortion. I have changed my mind since writing this piece and no longer see patients seeking an abortion; a notice in the waiting room makes this clear. After writing the piece I came to realise that I was doing this counselling, not because it was any help to the patient, but because I felt pressure from my partners (pressure which they had never expressed) to see patients wanting an abortion.

Then come some essays which were occasional pieces. These are generally a much easier read. "Thisness and quiddity" and "The human condition" might be good places for a reader to start." Darwin's dream", already mentioned, is a short story that encapsulates the advances in evolutionary theory relating to altruism that have occurred between the writing of "Beyond altruism" in 2001 and the present day.

There follow some pieces on teaching "Evidence based medicine", and then some connected to work I used to do as a medical examiner at "Freedom from Torture," formerly "The medical foundation for the care of victims of torture" The penultimate group are some rather disparate talks and articles on medicine and society included simply to illustrate my belief that a General Practitioner should be engaged with the society in which he works. These pieces and those connected to care for refugees are also related to the title of the book, "General Practice as if people mattered" but in a different way. These are the people, refugees, the terminally ill and unborn children who do not matter to society, yet society is judged by its care for them, as Rabi Hugo Gryn reminded us[3]. The final link with the title is that the NHS was set up to treat people. When my generation started work in the NHS, we considered only the need of the person in front of us, not their entitlement. In recent years there has been a campaign, led by governments, for an NHS that treats only UK citizens and not other people, not for example, "refused asylum seekers". I campaigned with many others against this change, and this is reflected in the section containing articles on refugees and asylum seekers.

The last piece is an autobiographical fragment. None of the pieces in this collection have been rewritten; were I to rewrite the initial three I would give more place to the physical body; as we age we can no longer take it for granted. Many of these pieces first appeared in the college journal (the BJGP). I am grateful to them for permission to republish these pieces. I soon learnt the word

---

[3] I believe that the line our society will take in this matter on how you are to people to whom you owe nothing is a signal. It is the critical signal that we give to our young and I hope and pray that it is a test we shall not fail." Rabi Hugo Gryn, see page 126 in this book.

"God" was taboo in the BJGP and tended to be edited out. I much enjoyed smuggling it in where possible.

In this introduction it is time to make it explicit that I am a Christian. However, my purpose in almost all these pieces, to booster the morale of my fellow general practitioners by showing that our job is worth both thinking about seriously and doing well, remains unchanged.

A proposed theoretical framework

The following three papers, of which two were published in the BJGP, are linked. They provide a theoretical framework for primary care. They were written in the years after my MSc in General Practice at King's college. In the oral examination at the end of the degree the external examiner asked me if the course had changed my view of the world. I could not give a pat answer then, but now I would say that my view had changed from seeing people as primarily individuals to seeing them more as social beings, as poised, indeed, on the cusp between being an individual and a social being.

What are the limits of natural science as applied to medicine?
Br J Gen Pract. 2002 Oct; 52(483): 870–871.

Introduction
By natural science I mean the traditional methods of physics, chemistry and biology as applied to medicine, the methods of what might be called reductionist science. In this essay I wish to explore the proper limits of these methods, and what effect using these methods will have on how we perceive the world. Is this relevant to general practice? I suggest that it is. For example, last night on call one lady rang twelve times to tell the duty doctor that she could not sleep. Do we really believe that applying these scientific methods - measuring, perhaps, her cerebral serotonin level - is going to provide a complete explanation? Maybe looking at her purely through a scientific mind-frame is going to blind us to her genuine distress, distress that is, admittedly, being expressed inappropriately. It is also true that our consulting rooms are frequently occupied with patients with "chronic multiple functional somatic symptoms" as recently reviewed in the BMJ (Bass & May 2002), patients whom scientific medicine from the primary to the tertiary level has failed to help, or even harmed.

The application of the scientific method to medicine leads first to wonder at what it can achieve, followed often by disillusion as to what it leaves out. It has been clear from the beginning that what it specifically excludes is any consideration of meaning. This is what George Herbert (Herbert 1995) explains in the following poem written in 1663, when scientific methods were "the new philosophy"[4]. He describes the sense of wonder scientific discoveries can bring, followed by disillusion as we become aware of the limitations of science.

> "Philosophers have measured mountains,
>
> Fathomed the depth of seas, of states, of kings,
>
> Walked with a staff to heaven and traced fountains:
> But there are two vast and spacious things,
>
> The which to measure it doth more behove,
>
> Yet there are few that sound them; sin and love."

"The Agony" (1633).

He is saying that natural science, while it can do marvellous things, cannot capture concepts to do with meaning and purpose in life (love and sin v.6). The same point is made by an excellent recent article comparing quantitative and qualitative research (Giacomini 2001).

Qualitative and quantitative research compared

Those methodologies that do look at meaning have since been called qualitative, as opposed to quantitative methods that are based on what I am calling natural science. These qualitative methods have quite different philosophical underpinnings than natural science, but what they share with each other is an acknowledgement of the importance of the observer in what is observed, and agreement that this needs to be recorded. Moreover, qualitative researchers, typically social scientists, differ from natural scientists in that they

---

[4] It might be noted here that it was George Herbert who first translated Bacon from the original Latin into English.

may not aspire to give a complete and self-consistent explanation of all reality, but are willing to use a range of methodologies to shed light on the same phenomenon. To borrow terms from the literary criticism of Mikhail Bakhtin the discourse of qualitative methods can be called a "polyphonic" discourse, that is to say it contains many distinct voices that, to some degree, recognise each other's validity. Scientific discourse based on quantitative methods by contrast is "monologizing", that is it recognises only one legitimate discourse and reduces all other voices to its own (Bakhtin 1997), (Puustinen 2000). Scientific discourse seeks to provide a complete and self-coherent explanation of reality. For this reason, while the various subjects which make up the social sciences are willing to interact, dialogue with them can be threatening to traditional scientists as it is at odds with their monologizing discourse about reality. The discourse of our patients also is typically polyphonic; that is to say that they happily engage in discourse with the pharmacist, the natural healer and the doctor, without feeling that any one of these is exclusive. It is only some doctors, educated into the monologizing discourse of science, who are disturbed by this, and lay claim to an exclusive perception of reality.

While scientists will readily acknowledge that they have not yet produced an exclusive and self-coherent explanation of reality, the claim is that it will be produced some day. Indeed the philosopher of science Thomas Kuhn (Kuhn 1970) claims that when one set of self-consistent explanations, which he calls a paradigm, wears thin, then scientists simply choose a new set of such explanations. Thus, he would claim that Newtonian physics was one paradigm, and that it was abandoned in favour of Einstein's theory of relativity.

The limitations of qualitative methods and quantitative methods can be compared by the following analogy. Qualitative research can be likened to "looking through a glass darkly" (I Cor. 13:12). This phrase of St Paul's refers to the ancients' use of a polished metal surface as a mirror. If you do this you will be aware not only of your reflection but also of the reflecting surface itself, which by its imperfections makes itself visible. Similarly, in qualitative research it is important to convey both what is seen and the perspective or "bias" of the researcher. In this way the fact that the research is an interpretation of the world is made explicit. Quantitative or natural science research can then to be likened to using a modern mirror. A modern mirror gives the viewer an illusion that they are seeing something "real". Yet this reality has a flaw hidden at its centre. In the case of the mirror this flaw is the reversal of handedness in every image, indeed every molecule seen in the mirror. The very perfection of the modern mirror makes it difficult to notice that the image is radically different from reality. The flaws hidden in natural science are equally hidden and equally pervasive.

The flaws or limitations of natural science

There are at least three flaws or limitations. Firstly meaning is excluded from scientific discourse, yet most of us believe that it is crucial to understanding human beings ((MacIntyre 1985) p.81 quoting (Quine 1960) chapter 6)). Secondly natural science as applied to medicine is considered to be independent of the observer, even though this is not the case for Einstein's theory of special or general relativity. Thirdly natural science depends on the explicit hypothesis that reality can be completely described by a set of self-consistent axioms, an assumption that has been shown to be false by Gödel. The traditional scheme was that medical science would be based on the physical sciences, the physical sciences on mathematics, and mathematics on logic. To logic itself the "axiomatic method" would be applied in which, from a few well-chosen axioms, the whole corpus of knowledge could be derived purely from internal deduction without reference to anything else. This project is implicit in the school science curriculum. It is explicitly followed by Bertrand Russell in his "Principia Mathematica" (Whitehead & Russell 1927), or, on a more popular level, by Steven Hawkin in "A Brief History of Time" (Hawkin 1995) where he describes the search for a grand unifying theory. Yet we have known since Gödel's theorem (1931) (Gödel 1992) (Nagel & Newman 1959) that an axiomatic system's consistency cannot be proved within the system itself. Even more startlingly Gödel showed that however many axioms you use there will be statements which are true but cannot be demonstrated from those axioms. For example, it is easy to see by trial and error that each whole number is the sum of two primes, yet no mathematician has yet demonstrated this by the axiomatic method. This could be an example of a simple truth about the system of whole numbers that cannot be demonstrated from the axioms of this system. So Gödel is showing that while science can clearly give a good description of reality, it is giving one whose consistency cannot be proven and which is demonstrably incomplete.

Conclusion

The very success of modern science blinds us to the fact that it only another description of reality, and moreover one which systematically excludes meaning, often fails to take into account the effect of the observer on what he observes and is demonstrably both improvable and incomplete. To lay out the limitations of natural science as applied to health is not to decry its use. On the contrary it has proved a startlingly useful way of understanding reality. To use it correctly, however, it is necessary to have an idea of its limitations.

References

Bakhtin, M. 1997, *Problems in Dostoyevsky's poetics* University of Minnesota Press, Minneapolis.

Bass, C. & May, S. 2002, "ABC of psychological medicine: Chronic multiple functional somatic symptoms", *BMJ*, vol. 325,no. 7359, pp. 323-326.

Giacomini, M. 2001, "The rocky road: qualitative research as evidence", *Evidence-Based Medicine*, vol. 6,no. 1, pp. 4-5.

Gödel, K. 1992, *On formally undecidable propositions in Principia Mathematica and related systems* Dover publications, London.

Hawkin, S. 1995, *A Brief History of time* Bantam, London.

Herbert, G. 1995, *George Herbert; The Complete English Works* David Campbell Publishers Ltd., London.

Kuhn, T. 1970, *The structure of scientific revolutions* University of Chicago Press, Chicago.

MacIntyre, A. 1985, *After Virtue*, 2nd edn, Duckworth, London.

Nagel, E. & Newman, J. 1959, *Gödel's proof* Routledge, Kegan and Paul, London.

Puustinen, R. 2000, "Voices to be heard - the many positions of a physician in Anton Chekhov's short story, "A case history"", *J.Med.Ethics*, vol. 26, pp. 37-42.

Quine, W. 1960, *Word and Object*.

Whitehead, A. & Russell, B. 1927, *Principia Mathematica* Cambridge University Press, Cambridge.

Consultation analysis "after Bakhtin"

The consultation has been analysed many different ways. It is possible to apply the literary criticism of Bakhtin, designed initially for the novel, to the consultation. Two basic categories need to be grasped. He applies the term "monologizing discourse" to any scheme of ideas that attempts to give a full description of reality without referring to concepts outside itself. Natural science, some forms of Marxism and Roman Catholicism are monologizing discourses. The scientific paper is a literary example, and the presentation on a grand round, an oral one. Such a discourse necessarily simplifies and excludes. At the extreme such a discourse will distort reality so that "to a hammer everything looks like a nail", or to give another example; "to a manufacturer of

10

Prozac everything looks like depression". A polyphonic discourse is one where many different voices giving different and often contradictory accounts of reality exist simultaneously in a person's head. Such is the normal condition for many people who will happily use concepts from homeopathy, conventional medicine and, say, Yoga, to help them deal with the world. It is, for Bakhtin, the normal form of the novel.

Some general practice consultations can then be seen, by the doctor or the patient, as an attempt to force the polyphonic discourse of the patient into the monologizing discourse of science. The following fictional consultation is analysed according to this scheme.

Patient. "I've got a terrible headache these days. My wife says I'm stressed out from all the hours I do at work."

(Wife's voice, explanation based on "stress" model.)

Doctor. "Mmmm."

Patient. "I've also got this knot at the back of my neck. My osteopath says that my neck is misaligned, and my headache gets better every time he treats me."

(Osteopath's voice, explanation based on osteopathy.)

Doctor. "Anything else happening?"

Patient. "Since my mum died four months ago, as well as the headache I've felt down and not enjoyed anything. I dream about her telling me I've been a naughty boy and wake up in a terrible sweat."

(Mother's voice, explanation based on guilt and dreams. The patient has so far shared three different explanatory systems.)

Doctor. "So you've been feeling stressed and down with a headache since your mother died. You've got all the symptoms of a reactive depression. The chemicals in your brain are low. You will get better with these anti-depressant tablets I'm going to give you. They will return the chemicals to their normal levels."

(Monologizing discourse seeking to explain all the ideas so far elicited by one scheme of "scientific" thought.)

Patient. "That's great doctor. But can I carry on with the osteopath and my natural healing tablets from the chemist as well?"

(Patient resists the doctor's monologizing discourse and places it instead as merely an extra voice in his polyphonic world.)

The consultation can be seen, then, as an attempt to listen to the "novel" of the patient's world and recast it according to the rules of scientific discourse. This transformation both requires great skill and is impossible. It requires great skill because the doctor must be familiar with both the patient's language and that of science. It is impossible because ultimately the monologizing discourse cannot capture the richness of a polyphonic world.

"What is man?"
Br J Gen Pract. 2003;53(491):504–505.

We do not come into this world with any labels attached. Man is to himself a mysterious creation. This question is the old question about the nature of man, in which, as men, we all have an understandable interest. The psalmist asks God,

"What is man, that you are mindful of him,

 Yet you have made him a little less than a God?"

Ps 8;4-6

The psalmist ponders the question of man's nature. He finds him awkwardly placed between insignificance and near divinity. The same is true today. One minute, in the consultation, it seems as if a wonderful power of sympathy and understanding is flowing through me, yet the next minute in the coffee room I can get thoroughly upset over some minute or imagined slight.

How we understand man has a big effect on what we see of him, and therefore how we treat him. Some people hold an unquestioned model of man, the model which they learnt as they grew up. Such people can be thrown as they realise that other people hold a quite different model. This realisation can be brought about by studying sociology or psychology, by meeting other cultures [1], or simply by the infinite variety of general practice. It can be a re-assurance to realise that only certain models of man are in general use in our culture. The following three models might be held, to some degree, to classify most of the models available to us.

1) Rational man, man as an individual man,
2) Social man, man as primarily a member of a group,
3) and Religious man, man seen primarily in relation to a creator.
Each model finds its adherents in contemporary European culture.

1) Rational man. This is probably the dominant model now, especially in academic circles. It can be described as follows. Man is seen as a rational individual. He chooses his actions by deciding what is best for him from his individual point of view. Society is seen simply as an aggregation of pre-existing individuals. This is how Hobbes saw society [2].

This picture of rational self-interest as a dominant force has built up slowly. Where La Rochefoucauld [3] emphasised that apparent altruism was often hidden self-interest, Hume [4] saw self-interest as one among many motivations. That flower of the Scottish enlightenment, Adam Smith, did not see man as purely rational, but appealed to rational self-interest as a protection against man's pride[5]. Only when we reach Bentham [6] or Nietzsche do we find philosophers who held that altruism could not exist, and all was self-interest. This emergence is well described by MacIntyre's "A short history of ethics" [7]. This model of rational man is that of most cotemporary economics and some political science. It has proved an excellent model where there is a possibility of quantifying, and it has shed light on many aspects of human behaviour. However, it finds it difficult to account for the possibility of man's co-operation because each man is seen as making his own self-interested decision. Altruism is seen by some as a disconfirming case for the "rational man" model. A true believer in rational man theory, once he accepts that altruistic motives occur, albeit rarely, he has to admit of the existence of a world beyond the perceptions of his previous "view-of-the-world". Indeed this is explicitly the journey taken by Monroe [8] and Batson (a social psychologist) [9] in their rather different books on altruism. Driven to extremes the "rational man" view leads to an extremely poor picture of man whose ultimate logic is depicted by WH Auden in "The shield of Achilles" [10].

"That girls are raped,

that two boys knife a third,

Were axioms to him, who'd never heard

Of any world where promises are kept,

Or one could weep because another wept."

Auden is pointing out that if there is only self-interest and no trust, then it will be a bleak world indeed in which we live.

The difficulties this model presents have been well described by Hardin's "tragedy of the commons where the cows overgraze land held in common [11]. A whole volume of essays bringing together current criticism of this model from contemporary economics, politics and psychology has been published [12]. There have been two contemporary developments of this picture. According to Ogden [13] psychological theory has come from seeing man as a passive responder to stimuli to seeing him as an active appraiser of risk, first in the environment, and increasingly within his own self. Giddens [14] has described post-modern man as defining himself by the choices he makes. By this he means, for example, that I choose my food in order to define and declare who I am, rather than eating what is normal or thought suitable for my state in life.

2) The social model of man. In this model a person is defined by his position in society. He is, as it were, constituted by the rights, duties and norms of his position. It is a familiar model to anyone who attended a public school. The essential facts about a boy are stated by his position in the school hierarchy, not by his personal choices. A boy is defined by being, let us say, a fifth year boy in a certain house with certain privileges and duties. If one knows this, then nothing else is worth knowing about him. His thoughts and actions, indeed where he is at any moment of the day can be confidently predicted just from this knowledge. In a similar way Marxists believed that a man's essential being was determined by his economic position in society, his social class. This was the structure. Anything else, his religion, his opinions, was called the super-structure and could be determined from it. An analogy can be made with language. Language does not exist in the absence of human beings, yet it precedes the existence of the individual. Language moulds and limits the ways individuals can think. The same may be said of the rules of society. (This is one of the insights of the structuralists [15]). Certain goods, especially money, have no "objective" existence, but are essentially "social" goods [16]. Within this model altruism is not a problem. Both altruism and "rational self-interest" are seen as alternative social norms. Yet this model can be taken too far and lead to the dreadful totalitarian excesses of Nazism and communism both Russian and Chinese. The engineered famines of Stalin in the Ukraine in the 1930s and Mao in China in 1958 spring to mind. This last famine, engineered by man, caused many more deaths than World War II [17].

3) Finally, "religious man" is man defined primarily by his relation to a creator. Belief in a creator is common to most but not all cultures. If a creator exists then one's relation to him is of great importance. Even if we just think he might exist; the stakes are so high that we may be wiser to bet that he does exist. This insight is known as "Pascal's wager" after Pascal, the founder of modern probability theory, who first set it out[18]. However exclusive attention to this relationship with the creator also leads to an impoverished picture of man. In the following passage Thomas Merton, who as a Trappist monk was vowed to a lifetime of

poverty and silence, in this passage opposes an exclusively "vertical" relationship with God;

"For it is the survival of religion as an abstract formality without a humanist matrix, religion apart from man …religion without any human epiphany in art, in work, in social forms: this is what is killing religion in our midst today, and not atheists [19]." It was men who believed that only the vertical relationship with God was important who were responsible for the inquisition and for mankind's innumerable wars of religion. From this perspective, if only man's relationship with God is important, then one can justify "killing a man in order to save his soul".

In a previous article I contrasted a polyphonic discourse (one where several different models are heard with mutual respect) to a monologizing discourse which believes one model holds the full and exclusive truth [20]. This, I believe is our situation with these models of man. Each can tell us something about him, but if any one is taken exclusively, as a monologizing discourse, it leads to danger. Initially it leads to blindness about things outside the model. For example, in the models above, rational man cannot perceive altruism, social man devalues personal beliefs, and an exclusively religious perspective fails to perceive the value of social life. Eventually a monologizing discourse can lead to tyranny, first to a state organised only for people who are willing to fit in with a certain understanding of man, leading sometimes to a state which sponsors torturers to stretch or chop people until they fit into, or accept the validity of, their scheme. For example, in the models above, the rational man model can lead to unbridled liberal economics, the social model can lead to the totalitarian state, and the exclusively religious model to religious persecution. Different models of man also lead to different therapeutic possibilities, as beautifully explained by the psychiatrist and philosopher Patrick Bracken in the case of post-traumatic stress disorder (PTSD)[21].

There is one final distinction to make. To say each insight into the nature of man is partial is not to commit oneself to the philosophical position that there is no objective truth. It is equally compatible with the position that there is an objective truth which may be partially grasped in a number of different ways.

Reference List

1. Shweder R, Bourne E. Does the concept of person vary cross-culturally? In Marsella A, Bourne E, eds. *Cultural conceptions of mental health and therapy*, Dordrecht: Reidel, 1982.

2. Hobbes T. Leviathan; or the matter form and power of a commonwealth, ecclesiastical and civil. London: A. Crooke, 1651.

3. La Rochefoucauld F. Moral maxims and reflections, in four parts. London: Gillyflower, Sare, & Everingham, 1691.

4. Hume A. A treatise of human nature. Oxford: Oxford University Press, 1739.

5. Holmes S. The secret history of self-interest. In Mansbridge J, ed. *Beyond self-interest*, pp 267-86. Chicago: University of Chicago Press, 1990.

6. Bentham J. An introduction to the principles of morals and legislation. Oxford: The Clarendon Press, 1789.

7. MacIntyre A. A short history of ethics. London: Routledge, 1998.

8. Monroe KR. The heart of altruism: perceptions of a common humanity. Princeton, New Jersey: Princeton University Press, 1996.

9. Batson C. The altruism question: towards a social psychological answer. New Jersey: Lawrence Erlbaum Associates, Inc., 1991.

10. Auden WH. Collected Poems. London: Faber and Faber, 1976.

11. Hardin G. The tragedy of the commons. *Science* 1968;**162**:1243-8.

12. Mansbridge J.J. Beyond self-interest. University of Chicago Press: Chicago, 1990.

13. Ogden J. Psychological theory and the creation of the risky self. *Social Science and Medicine* 1995;**40**:409-15.

14. Giddens A. The consequences of modernity. Cambridge: Polity Press, 1991.

15. Lévi-Strauss C. Tristes Tropiques. Paris: Librairie Plon, 1955.

16. Taylor, C. Irreducibly social goods. 1989. Canberra, Australian National University. Proceedings of the conference on Rationality, Individuality and Public Policy.

Ref Type: Conference Proceeding

17. Smil V. China's great famine Forty years later. *BMJ* 1999;**319**:1619-21.

18. Pascal B. Pensees. London: Penguin, 1970. pensee number 418 (Krailsheimer number)

19. Merton T. The hidden ground of love. New York: Farrar Strauss Giroux, 1985.

20. Vernon J. The limitations of natural science as applied to medicine. *BJGP* 2002;**52**:870-1.

21. Bracken P. Trauma, culture, meaning and philosophy. London: Whurr publishers, 2002.

Consultation analysis; taking into account the patient's view of man

Roger Neighbour has taught us to pay attention to the patient's language in the consultation. He has stated that if we use the same language (visual, auditory or kinaesthetic) as the patient then he will understand us better. Doing this he is following the old adage "Go in at the patient's door and bring him out at your own".

Now the same applies to the patient's internal model of what a human being is. We should listen carefully to what the patient says and discern which model of man he is using. Then we can phrase our reply using the same model. In this way the patient is much more likely to feel that we are on his wavelength and follow our advice.

The following is an example. In this fictional consultation the doctor sees a seventy year old man with atrial fibrillation and a recent TIA. The doctor has decided to persuade his patient to go on warfarin.

Rational model of man

Patient: "Well, doctor, what does this irregular rhythm you've found mean for me? I do not want tablets, if possible, because there is always a risk of side-effects."

(Note the language of risk and of the individual point of view, so the doctor responds in kind)

Doctor: "Well you're quite right to think of it in terms of risks and benefits. The increased risk that this irregular heart rhythm brings is that of stroke. What does a stroke mean to you?"

Patient: "My mother had a terrible stroke and was in a home for years, I never want to be like that."

(The doctor is home and dry.)

Social model of man

Patient: "Doctor, tell me, what do people normally do for this irregular heart rhythm, I mean, what is the right thing to do?"

(Note the language of norms and rights, sounds like a social model of man.)

Doctor: "Professor Wright, our local geriatrician puts all his patients with this irregular rhythm on warfarin and that is what I recommend for you."

(Appeal to authority should go down well here.)

Religious model of man

Patient (a Roman Catholic priest): "Last night when I went to bed, my hand was numb and I could not move it. So I just prayed to God and when I woke up it was fine. Now you tell me I should take some tablets. Look if God wants to take me, I'm ready to go."

Doctor: "Now, father, we need to consider what God wants for you. Does he not want you to look after the parish a little longer?"

(Staying within model plus a little judicious flattery.)

These are the sort of verbal tactics that many general practitioners probably use without, perhaps, being fully aware of them. However, they are powerful tools, and should be used with respect for the patient, and not in order to manipulate him.

What is a General Practitioner? 2004

Written after the previous two pieces but never published, this piece re-iterates the previous two and attempts to relate them to the writings of earlier authors about General Practice; Lane, Huygens (a Dutch author who wrote a wonderful photo essay on the importance of family relations in his practice) and Berger (who wrote a wonderful photo essay about a rural GP, Dr Sassal). It also considers virtue ethics and narrative medicine. The new concept of the health care triangle is explored and the consequences of the 1990 and 2004 GP contracts turning GPs from providers of unbiased medical advice to paid providers of government provided medical advice are considered. Finally, continuity of care and narrative medicine are briefly examined.

This essay is emphatically not an attempt to define the core curriculum of General Practice, a worthy but entirely different enterprise. The core curriculum will differ from year to year and country to country. Here we are looking to see if anything, common across cultures, can define the first contact with a paid professional in the patient's journey from person to patient. In this essay, then, I am defining General Practice, or first contact primary care in general, not by its content, but by its context.

Many General Practitioners (GPs) in the United Kingdom today are uncertain about their role. A new contract (the 2004 GP contract) has been agreed and changes in their role seem to occur with ever increasing frequency. There are many sources for this uncertainty, which is not limited to General Practitioners or doctors. It is reflected in the BMJ themed issue last year called "What is a good doctor?" [1]. This uncertainty applies to all professions. Indeed, the whole of western society is said to have entered a state of post-modernity. This means a situation where everything is challenged and no single over-arching explanation of the world is held by most citizens [2]. There is an attack on the idea of the professions, especially the medical profession, unmasking the extent to which professionalism can be a cover for seeking power [3]. At a time of change people are asking; "What is a General

Practitioner/ Family Doctor?" In answer to this question, I wish to offer some general ideas, rather than a systematic approach, as a contribution to this debate.

The first point of contact

A first step might be to ask; "can any generalisations about primary care be made today?" While General Practice in the UK today is in a rapid state of flux, it remains a primary care speciality; that is one which is a point of first contact with the public. If any generalisations can be made about primary care today, they will apply to General Practitioners and continue do so as long as General Practitioners and Family Doctors have a frontline role. In his journey from being a person to becoming the patient, the potential patient will typically discuss his illness with a number of people such as friends or relatives [4] [5]. The distinguishing feature of the primary care worker is that he is the first paid point of contact.

The health care triangle

We can look at this from another angle. Most health care interactions can be analysed in terms of three players. The first player is the patient or client. The second player is the one who pays, typically in the UK, the state. The third player is the health care professional such as a General Practitioner who is paid for providing health care. Each player has separate interests and a separate perspective.

Patient

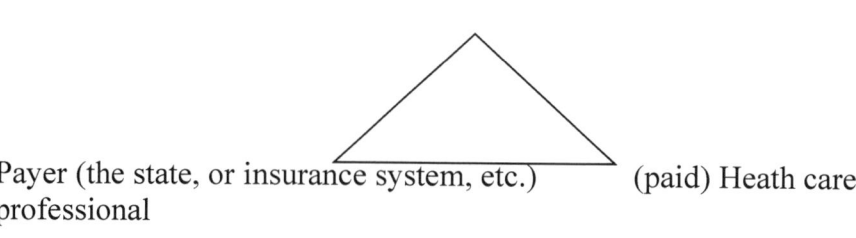

Payer (the state, or insurance system, etc.)   (paid) Heath care professional

The health care triangle

22

A systematic review of what patients want from general practice, for example, concluded that patients rate most highly the doctors' "humaneness" [6]. The state, on the other hand, will tend to talk in terms of cost effectiveness while doctors value competencies and communication skills. These different perspectives have been highlighted in recent articles in the BMJ [7] [8] and an accompanying editorial [9]. As explained above, what is specific about the encounter with the primary health care professional, however, is that it is the first encounter for which advice is paid.

It is worth looking at the health care triangle in a bit more detail. The primary health care triangle can be reduced to an interaction between two parties in a number of ways. For example, it may be that the patient pays in person, eliminating the state as a third party. This was the situation with patients in the 18th century when the rich patient paid the physician [10]. In this dyad the patient held much more power and could choose a physician with beliefs aligned to his.

Patient – also the payer -------------------------------- Health care professional

The health care triangle collapsed into a two-player system (a dyad)

In the health care triangle as currently constituted in Britain and some other European countries it is the one who pays, the state, which chooses the ideological basis of the medicine offered. The state chooses to pay for modern Western "scientific" medicine. The change from personal physician to payment by the state occurred gradually in the UK and was finalised with the advent of the NHS. General Practitioners working at this time of transition noticed the significance of the change. A General Practitioner author of the time Dr Kenneth Lane wrote; "He [the GP] has a duty to society not to waste public money. The duty to the patient has always been admitted….The duty to society developed suddenly with the coming of the National Health Service in 1948, and is being accepted slowly."[11].

So here are two generalisations about primary care which can be applied to general practice. The primary care physician is the first person to be paid to listen to the patient's story. The primary care physician is paid by the state – in Western cultures at least – to analyse the patient's story according the beliefs of Western scientific medicine. A subtle distinction emerged with the 1990 GP contract. General Practitioners used to be paid to provide the medical advice they thought best for the patient, comparable in the financial sector to an independent financial adviser. With the 1990 and new 2004 contracts General Practitioners will be largely paid to provide the advice that the government thinks is best. They will be, as it were, tied medical advisers – tied to the government's preferred scientific advice. There is nothing wrong with this, legally or morally, but it is a difference. It is a difference which patients will notice, as they already have over the MMR controversy [12] and which is likely to lead to an expanding market for private primary care.

Monologizing discourse and polyphonic discourse

Let us return to the question of scientific medicine applying in particular the work of the Russian philosopher and literary critic Mikhail Bakhtin [13] [14;15]. If we view scientific medicine as one of several possible discourses about the world, then a literary critic might help us to identify certain specific features of scientific discourse. According to Bakhtin there are some key differences between the scientific discourse in which doctors are trained and the stories that patients tell us. Turning their stories into our language is difficult and loses some of the message. As Dr. Kenneth Lane put it; "we fit patients into categories to suit our knowledge." These key differences between scientific discourse and patients' stories have an effect on the daily lives of all primary care workers. Bearing in mind Bakhtin's contribution these differences can be tabulated as shown below:

Differences between scientific discourse and the patient's discourse according to Bakhtin

	Scientific discourse	Patient's discourse
Bakhtin's terminology	Monologizing discourse	Polyphonic discourse
User believes discourse is potentially able to explain everything	Yes	No
User believes discourse is an exclusive explanation	Yes	No
User can use discourse simultaneously with a discourse based on different and incompatible beliefs	No	yes

To understand this table further we need to realise that positivists such as Comte believe that science can explain everything [16]. If it is pointed out to them that science has not explained everything, they will modify their stance to say that it will explain everything "one day". They also believe that only scientific explanations are true – from their point of view non-scientific explanations are by definition incorrect. This sort of discourse was called by Bakhtin "monologizing discourse". The view of many patients about their health beliefs is quite different. They may hold several and often quite incompatible health beliefs about the same symptoms and express them within a couple of minutes. For example, a mother might bring her daughter with a headache and within a couple of sentences offer the explanations that the headaches are due to the stress of the new school term and are due to an allergy to wheat in the food. They believe that different and mutually incompatible explanations can both be right. Patients, then, in Bakhtin's terminology, are using a polyphonic discourse.

Another way of putting this is to say that a general practitioner is an interpreter who turns the patient's polyphonic discourse into the monologizing discourse of science. More exactly this is involves not only interpreting (oral to oral) but an element of transcribing (oral to written). The general practitioner mediates between the oral and the written language, between the patient's polyphonic discourse and the monologizing discourse of science, and between the "lay views" of the patient (Helman) [17] and discourse dominant in that society (scientific medicine in our case).

Virtue ethics

Does this view of an essential element of general practice have any implications for the character and training of general practitioners? Virtue ethics is, in part, the study of which character is appropriate for a particular way of life. Virtue ethics were studied by Aristotle and Aquinas and revived in recent times by Alasdair McIntyre [18]. As McIntyre sees it, a certain way of life, like primary care (which he calls a practice), calls for certain virtues which suit one for that way of life. The call to establish which virtues suit general practice in an empirical way has been made before by Toon [19]. Some suitable practices can be deduced from the observations which have just been made. If a General Practitioner is, at least in part, an interpreter between two cultures, he needs to be familiar with both and act as an advocate for each to the other. So a primary care practitioner will seek to be familiar with both scientific medicine and the culture of the people he serves. This is not an argument that he should have less scientific medicine than his hospital colleagues – rather that he should know other things as well.

Secondly because the General Practitioner stands between the patient and the state he needs to earn the trust of both. As far as the patient is concerned this means he needs to be able to see the world through his eyes and feel his emotions; intellectual and emotional empathy. As far as the state is concerned this calls for honesty and straightforwardness in our dealings with the state. It also calls for a continuous attempt to engage with the state and improve the frequent reorganisations it imposes by keeping the good parts and amending the poor ones. So from our observations about primary care workers we can deduce something about the sort of things they should do and be, and something about their character. Similarly, one could deduce some implications for their training.

Continuity of care

Although I have not set out to provide a systematic answer to the question; "What is a General Practitioner?" there are some concepts that are too important just to omit. One of these is continuity of care. This is not a constitutive part of the role of a primary care worker as defined above. Yet many General Practitioners and patients do value it. Its importance has been particularly championed by a past president of the Royal College of General Practitioners of the UK, Professor Pereira-Grey [20;21]. Because of the long time scales involved the importance of continuity is difficult to demonstrate in an objective way and may well differ for different illnesses and different patients. An idea of the possible benefit of continuity of care can be gained from the classic book by John Berger about general practice "A Fortunate Man" [22]. Even more eloquent is Professor Huygen's "Family Medicine." [23] He looked after a small number of Dutch families from the 1940s to the 1970s. His thesis is that the family is a unit which contributes to the creation and expression of illness in the individual. He was an early exponent of family therapy in a general practice setting. More recently John Launer in his book and courses has adapted systems theory from family therapy to use in general practice [24]. He calls his book "Narrative-based medicine". This word narrative brings us to the last strand I wish to mention. This strand of "narrative medicine" originating in the USA [25] has been brought to the UK by Hurwitz and Greenhalgh [26]. There can be a temptation to impoverish the study of narrative by making each story equivalent in weight as if there was no objective truth. To consider each story as a partial description of an objective truth, bearing in mind the formal differences alluded to above between the patient's stories and the scientific one yields a more fruitful analysis. In conclusion general practitioners are heirs to a rich intellectual tradition, one which has to be reworked in every generation. Similarly, being a general practitioner is not something achieved once and for all, but rather challenged each day as I decide; "Do I actually go out and answer that urgent call?", and "Do I make the effort to listen attentively to the distressed patient in front of me?"

Reference List

1. Smith, R et al. What is a good doctor and how do you make one? BMJ 325. 28-9-2002.

Ref Type: Journal (Full)

2. Lyotard J. The postmodern condition: a report on knowledge. Manchester: Manchester University Press, 1979.

3. Friedson E. The profession of medicine. New York: Dodd, Mead and Company, 1970.

4. Mechanic D, .Volkart E. Illness behaviour and medical diagnosis. *Journal of health and human behaviour* 1960;**1**:86-94.

5. Zola I. Pathways to the doctor: from person to patient. *Social Science and Medicine* 1973;**7**:677-89.

6. Wensing M, Jung H, Mainz J, Olesen F, Grol R. A systematic review of the literature on patients' priorities for general practice care. Part 1: Description of the research domain. *Soc Sci Med* 1998;**47**:1573-88.

7. Wright EB, Holcombe C, Salmon P. Doctors' communication of trust, care, and respect in breast cancer: qualitative study. *BMJ* 2004;**328**:864-0.

8. Britten N. Patients' expectations of consultations. *BMJ* 2004;**328**:416-7.

9. Smith R. The teaching of communication skills may be misguided. *BMJ* 2004;**328**:0-g.

10. Jewson N. The disappearance of the sick-man from medical cosmology 1770-1870. *Sociology* 1976;**10**:225-44.

11. Lane K. The longest art. London: RCGP, 1969.

12. Vernon G. Immunisation policy; from compliance to concordance? *BJGP* 2003;**53**:399-404.

13. Bakhtin M. Problems in Dostoyevsky's poetics. Minneapolis: University of Minnesota Press, 1997.

14. Puustinen R. Voices to be heard - the many positions of a physician in Anton Chekhov's short story, "A case history". *J.Med.Ethics* 2000;**26**:37-42.

15. Vernon G. The limitations of natural science as applied to medicine. *BJGP* 2002;**52**:870-1.

16. Comte A. Cours de philosophie positive. Paris: Bachelier, 1830.

17. Helman C. "Feed a cold and starve a fever": folk models of infection in an English suburban community and their relation to medical treatment. *Culture, Medicine and Psychiatry* 1978;**2**:107-37.

18. MacIntyre A. After Virtue. London: Duckworth, 1985.

19. Toon P. The sovereignty of virtue. *BJGP* 2002;**52**:695.

20. Baker R, Mainous A, Gray DJP, Love M. Exploration of the relationship between continuity, trust in regular doctors and patient satisfaction with consultations with family doctors. *Scand J Prim Health Care* 2003;**21**:27-32.

21. Gray DJP. The Key to personal care. *J R Coll Gen Pract* 1979;**29**:666-78.

22. Berger J. A fortunate man. London: Allen Lane The Penguin Press, 1967.

23. Huygen F. Family Medicine; the medical life history of families. London: RCGP, 1990.

24. Launer J. Narrative-based primary care, a practical guide. Abingdon: Radcliffe Medical Press, 2002.

25. Brody H. Stories of sickness. Oxford: Oxford University Press, 2002.

26. Greenhalgh T, Hurwitz B. Narrative based medicine. London: BMJ books, 1998.

Longer articles

This first article was written as a result of Thursday afternoons spent in Cambridge University library researching this topic. An early draft was seen and much improved by Professor Nicky Britten who was then writing a series of articles for the BMJ on concordance in the usage of medication.

Immunisation policy; from compliance to concordance?

Br J Gen Pract. 2003 May; 53(490): 399–404.

Introduction

Mass immunisation for protection from infectious disease is generally acknowledged to be one of the outstanding achievements of modern medicine[1] and its benefits have been eloquently set out [2]. Yet it has recently come under public suspicion with large sections of the population turning away from pertussis vaccination in the 1980s [3] and more recently from triple vaccine MMR [4][5][6]. The significant fall in coverage, which led to a pertussis epidemic in the 1980s, has not been repeated on the same scale for MMR[7]. Similarly there has been resistance against hepatitis B vaccination in France based on the belief that it causes multiple sclerosis[8]. A campaign there was so successful that routine immunisation of adolescents was suspended in 1997 [9]. While an older generation can remember the infectious diseases, there is now a generation which has never seen measles let alone polio or smallpox. There is a much greater public distrust of medications in general and vaccines in particular, together with an increased awareness of side-effects. In such a climate it is proving difficult to maintain the high coverage needed for herd immunity. The editor of the BJGP, Dr. David Jewell, has suggested it is time for a new approach to the public, listening to the lay voice without an excessive dependence on experts [10]. Shortly after this article, perhaps as a coincidence, the Joint Committee on Vaccination and Immunisation agreed to appoint a lay member. This appointment has, however, so far been delayed[11]. Can we engage the public in the decisions about vaccination, paralleling the advocated move from compliance to concordance with regard to medication [12] [13]? Are medicine taking and acceptance of immunisation sufficiently similar for this to be a useful analogy (see table 1)? Can research tell us anything about how those who refuse immunisations think, and therefore how we might talk to them?

	Immunisation	medicine taking
Public act	yes	no
one-off or continuous	mostly one-off	continuous
Potential effect of decision on other community members	++	+
Legitimate public interest	+++	+
Altruistic component to action	often	slight
typical level of full acceptance/compliance	80% +	50% [14] [15]

Table 1: The differences between immunisation and medicine taking

The third world

In the third world, vaccination, first as the Expanded Programme on Immunisation (EPI), and more recently as the Global Alliance for Vaccines and Immunisations (GAVI) [16]has proved to be even more dramatically effective. Here immunisation, especially against measles, has lowered rates of childhood mortality. This effect has been seen even where living standards are falling. (This is in contrast to the developed world where McKeown [17] long ago showed, though some would qualify this[18], that declining mortality preceded immunisations and was due to other factors, such as public health improvements and rising living standards.) Yet, even in the third world, there has been resistance against vaccination. For example, in the Philippines, a rumour arose that tetanus toxoid vaccination was being used for family planning purposes. For this reason, it was strongly opposed by the pro-life Roman Catholic Church. The church was able to obtain a court order forbidding the Department of Health to continue giving the vaccination [19] [20].

Herd immunity, altruism and consent

The effectiveness of immunisation depends on two factors. It depends on personal immunity leading to some protection against infection. It also depends on herd immunity which prevents the infectious agent from circulating in the community and protects both the immunised and the unimmunised. The decision to immunise a child therefore may have an altruistic element, that is to say that there is an intention to benefit not only the child but also the whole community[21]. This altruistic element will be particularly marked for some vaccines, and absent for some, such as tetanus vaccine. For example, in the early days of pertussis vaccination in the UK, children above six months old were vaccinated, yet the principal beneficiaries of herd immunity were children from birth to six months. These young babies were the ones who were most at risk from pertussis. In another striking example in Japan, vaccinating schoolchildren against influenza was obligatory from 1977-1987. This was principally to provide indirect protection against influenza in elderly adults[22]. This altruistic element is of direct relevance to informed consent because, unless the woman is aware of it, her consent is not informed. Valid consent requires a sound mind, sufficient understanding and a free agreement[23]. Consent has been particularly emphasised in the US and more recently in the UK [24]. The importance of this altruistic element is clear because the damage to the community is rapid and obvious if immunisation rates fall. In the UK in 1974, for example, a report on the adverse effects of pertussis vaccine was taken up by the media [25]. This led to a fall in vaccine uptake to 30%, and then an epidemic of pertussis. It took a decade for immunisation uptake to return to previous levels[3].

The scope of research to date

In summarising research to date it is important to realise both the variety of research methods used and the very different groups of people who do not accept immunisation and among whom this research is carried out. A non-systematic search reveals data in many places, mainly social science databases, with only a minority indexed in Medline. Techniques range from narrative based methods (including historical research) [26 27 28 29 30 31 32], to qualitative[33 34 35 36 37 38] and quantitative methods[39 40 41 42] and finally epidemiology[3;43].

The groups interviewed range from those who refuse all immunisations[44] to those who accept only some[45 19 20;33 34 35 3] and finally those who accept the full immunisation programme[38]. There is a particular shortage of qualitative research on the last group. There is, therefore, scope for research on why parents who have their children fully immunised choose to do so. Finally, the researchers set out to find very different sorts of reasons for refusal to immunise. Some researchers were looking for group reasons for refusal to immunise[44 46 19 20], others for individual reasons for refusal to immunise [33 34 35 36 37 44] and yet others were looking for difficulties of access due to geographical factors, transport or staff rudeness[47].

Research in the UK

Early research into vaccine coverage emphasised social and cultural factors such as class and employment [39] [40] [48]. Qualitative research in the UK into how people think about immunisation is sparse. An early qualitative paper showed that non-immunisers did not differ from immunisers so much in access to immunisation, as in their beliefs about immunisation[33]. In the 1980s Rogers and Pilgrim [34] [49] conducted a number of interviews with parents and professional groups. They emphasised that anti-immunisers had a rational position, albeit different from the official one. They noted, "This group of mothers tended to be paragons of virtue, if not zealots, about reducing potential risks to their children's health in every respect except immunisation". They also felt that the official view minimised or glossed over the possible side-effects of vaccines. These conclusions were criticised in other papers in the same symposium as Rogers and Pilgrim. These papers emphasised the safety of vaccines, the severity of some infectious diseases and the lack of evidence of long term harm from vaccines.[50].

Two UK papers have visited this area recently. The first was a focus group study with groups of both immunisers and non-immunisers [38]. This study, among the first to concentrate on immunisers, showed that they shared the concerns of non-immunisers. Non-immunisers were more likely to be concerned about unknown long-term side-effects of vaccines, and to consider that vaccines placed stress on the immune system rather than strengthening it [36]. The other UK study was of non-immunising parents [35]. In both studies the risk of side effects was found to be an important issue for the parents. They discussed immunisation from a risk perspective and had lost trust in health professionals. For these parents the decision about immunisation was an on-going process, not a single decision [37]. While immunisers felt that it would be their responsibility if their child developed an illness due to their failure to immunise, non-immunising parents took the opposite perspective. They would have felt guilty if their child had side-effects, but if their child fell ill this was seen as natural and not their responsibility [38] [34;51].

Research world-wide

There has been an organised effort by the WHO (the social science and immunisation project) to obtain data from developed and developing countries[52;53]. The results have been summarised by Streefland [8;47]. The causes of failure to immunise have been found to differ in developed and developing countries[8]. In developing countries non-immunisers may find access difficult, they may have had experience of rudeness from immunisation services, or they may belong to a social group whose ideology clashes with that of the government promoting the immunisation programme [54]. In developed countries resistance may be because of an organised belief system (homeopathy [55], Christian science [44], or anthroposophy [56]), but more typically it is on an individual basis, as a personal choice. Where there is individual choice, however, it may be informed by various sources. As well as the popular press and books, there are a plethora of websites which are violently against immunisation[57 58 59 60].

Streefland, in an excellent paper which summarises work to date on the sociology of immunisation, describes five explanatory perspectives on immunisation[47] (see table 2). Each perspective could be seen as a separate discourse, that is, a scheme of mutually coherent and related ideas. Any individual is likely to view the situation from more than one perspective or, if you will, participate in more than one discourse.

Table 2: Overleaf
Streefland's five perspectives explaining
differences in immunisation coverage [47]

Explanatory perspectives	Name of perspective	Whose perspective	Example
The perspective of variation in rational vaccine use	Group thinking	parents as members of a culture, medical anthropologists	"We Tumbuka people believe needles strengthen our children."
The perspective of collective decision by vaccination users	Normality	parents as members of a group	"We have our children immunised because it is the normal thing to do."
The perspective of trust in the competent provider	Trust	individual mother	"I have my child immunised because I trust the advice of this professional, whom I know."
The perspective of risk perception	Rational choice	individual mother	"I make a rational decision and I choose for my child on the basis of my perception of the risks and benefits."
The perspective of state, power	Public health	policy makers, epidemiologists,	"The protection

and the body	perspective	etc.	individuals gain from herd immunity is greater than individual immunity and therefore it is society's responsibility to ensure that children are immunised."

One perspective is that of normality; the mother who has her child immunised because it is the "normal" thing to do so. It is what her friends are doing, what her mother did to her and so on. Another is the discourse of the "rational agent". The mother decides what is best for the child based on her perception of the risks and benefits. This is the model which underlies psychological theories about health related behaviour, both the health belief model, [41;61] and protection motivation theory [62] [42]. This discourse feeds into the wider discourse in our society where our identity is defined by the choices we make as described by Anthony Giddens [63]. This perspective is that of the well-educated non-immunisers interviewed by Rogers and Pilgrim[49]. It contrasts with pre-modern societies where the group to which we belong more closely defines the choices that we make. However social factors still have strong effects in modern societies[64], indeed they have been recently shown to influence MMR coverage[65].

For the mother using the "rational choice" perspective the question of trust becomes important. Which source of information should she trust? The falling trust in experts is a recurring theme in modern society[66]. In the case of immunisation there is the particular problem that GPs no longer give unbiased advice. Rather, since the 1990 and 2004 contracts, they are paid by the

NHS to give the advice reckoned to be of greatest good to the community. Initially paying GPs to reach certain targets by improving their organisation and the advice they gave had dramatic results in improving immunisation coverage in the UK, although a Cochrane review of target payments world-wide shows only a small effect[67]. Some research suggests that non-immunising mothers are now discounting their GPs advice because they believe it is biased by his financial stake in the process [35] [38]. If this is the case then we should reconsider this method of payment.

How to improve coverage

Are there any other ways to improve coverage? There has been a recent leader in the BJGP [68], a Cochrane review showing the effectiveness of patient reminders[69] and a meta-analysis of interventions to improve immunisations [70]. These have shown that, after health service factors, financial incentives to mothers and reminders to mothers are the most effective interventions. Incentives to the mother have not been tried in the UK, but have been elsewhere. Proof of immunisation has been required for school entry in the USA, some parts of Germany and some states in Australia. In France proof of immunisation has been a prerequisite for receiving certain benefits[49].

What might we mean by concordance?

Concordance in immunisation policy must mean a process which occurs not only at the individual level, but also at a societal level. Concordance needs to be more than just a transfer of information about consumers' wishes to the state; it must involve to some degree a transfer of power. Simply improving presentation by means of techniques, such as focus groups to elicit opinion, might improve coverage in the short term but could be seen in the longer term as coercing the public and thus further alienate them. This potential danger of the abuse of qualitative methods has recently been pointed out[71]. Concordance in immunisation policy is a specific example of the question of involving the public in health care decisions. According to Holm we can only hope to make this process transparent, accountable and fair [72]. We cannot hope to make it fully rational because the goals of a health care system are multiple and fuzzy. The problem with immunisation is how to capture the multiple explanatory discourses used by the parties involved, especially the mothers, and make them mutually comprehensible[73;74]. This does not necessarily mean something warm and cosy. For example, if the day came when most mothers thought of immunisation in terms of risk analysis, then the current successful policy of immunising baby boys against rubella would become untenable because there is little benefit to the individual boy.

Concordance must mean more than "evidence-based health care"[75] simplistically interpreted. Those who pioneered evidence based medicine emphasized from the beginning that the evidence should be applied to an individual[76]. However, some of those who followed their lead have not taken into account that many people look at life quite happily from a number of different perspectives. For example, they may look at life both from a scientific view of the world, and from other and quite incompatible world views. Concordance, then, should mean not only applying the evidence to the individual but also dialogue between perspectives based on different views of the world. It means an exchange of views and mutual respect between these very different views. Certainly, this can be difficult. For example the recent report of the CMO's working party on CFS/ME[77] attempted to synthesise disparate voices but failed to keep the original broad-based membership together .

That it may be possible is, however, at least suggested by an interesting new approach has been pioneered by Professor Jake Chapman, working with large organisations [78]. He maintains that large organisations, and the immunisation system would be one, are not simple linear systems that can be managed by a command and control style of management. Rather they are complex adaptive systems, whose whole is, in some sense, greater than the sum of its parts. His approach, which has been successful with large government IT projects[79], involves finding solutions to which all participants subscribe, sensitivity to different perspectives, and avoiding multiple pre-set targets which can have perverse effects.

Conclusion

There have been protests against immunisation from the earliest days of smallpox vaccinations[26] [27] [28] [29] [31]. In a free society it has proved necessary to allow for conscientious objection and accept less than 100% coverage. However, in our current post-modern society the "top-down" policy currently pursued by the Department of Health is, in the opinion of many, likely to work less and less well. We will need to engage with the public concerning the need for immunisation, perhaps by means of focus groups to elicit public opinion and go beyond the public surveys currently carried out [80]. We will need better public information campaigns. (Some videos already exist and these could be more widely disseminated[81-83]). Perhaps the government's new health promotion agency will be the right agency to organise this[84]. There needs to be a shift in immunisation practice parallel to that in taking medicines from compliance to concordance. Such a change requires on-going qualitative research into how both immunisers and non-immunisers think. It will require much greater funds for public information campaigns when new immunisations are decided upon. But such changes are needed if the benefits of this old and established public health practice are to be maintained in the new millennium. It could be said that public policy about immunisation illustrates and reflects a current tension in wider health policy between an increased reliance on scientific evidence and a wish to have a patient centred approach, and between the needs as defined by the experts and the wants expressed by the public.

The latest change in the UK immunisation policy against diphtheria is a good example of the current approach. There have been epidemics of diphtheria in the countries of the old Soviet Union. Surveys have shown that the adult population of the UK have little protection against diphtheria[85]. The response of the Department of Health has been to write to vaccine manufacturers in the UK discouraging them from producing single antigen tetanus vaccine. Soon only double antigen tetanus and diphtheria vaccine will be available. A circular has been sent to GPs and casualty departments informing them of this change[85]. There has been no consultation or attempt to inform the public. It will be left to GPs and others to inform patients at the time they attend us with minor injuries. This approach is open to the risk that another anti-vaccine movement will arise demanding single tetanus vaccine. A new approach that elicited public opinion, allowed for conscientious objection, involved the target groups in decision making, and included a public information campaign which created a social demand for immunisation [47 54 86] would reduce these risks.

With acknowledgements to Professor Nicky Britten for her helpful suggestions.

Reference List

1. Poland G, Murray D, Bonilla-Guerrero R. Science, medicine, and the future: New vaccine development. *BMJ* 2002;**324**:1315-9.

2. Bedford H,.Elliman D. Concerns about immunisation. *BMJ* 2000;**320**:240-3.

3. Gangarosa E, Galazka A, Wolfe C, Phillips L, Gangarosa R, Miller E *et al*. Impact of anti-vaccine movements on pertussis control: the untold story. *Lancet* 1998;**351**:356-61.

4. Elliman D,.Bedford H. MMR vaccine - worries are not justified. *Arch Dis Child* 2001;**85**:271-4.

5. Bedford H,.Elliman D. Private eye special report on MMR. *BMJ* 2002;**324**:1224.

6. Wakefield A, Murch S, Anthony A, Casson D, Malik M. Ileal-lymphoid nodular hyperplasia, non-specific colitis, and pervasive developmental disorder in children. *Lancet* 1998;**351**:1327-8.

7. Ramsay M, Yarwood J, Lewis D, Campbell H, White J. Parental confidence in measles, mumps and rubella vaccine: evidence from vaccine coverage and attitudinal surveys. *BJGP* 2003;**52**:912-6.

8. Streefland P. Public doubts about vaccination safety and resistance against vaccination. *Health Policy* 2001;**55**:159-72.

9. Lack of evidence that hepatitis B causes multiple sclerosis. *Weekly epidemiological record* 1997;**72**:149-56.

10. Jewell D. MMR and the age of unreason. *BJGP* 2001;**51**:875-6.

11. Minutes of the Joint committee on vaccination and immunisation Jan 2002 http://www.doh.gov.uk/jcvi/mins25jan02.htm. 2002.

12. Royal pharmaceutical society of Great Britain. From compliance to concordance. Achieving shared goals in medicine taking. London: RPSGB, 1997.

13. Compliance to concordance www.concordance.org. 2002.

14. Haynes R, McDonald H, Montague P. Interventions for helping patients to follow prescriptions for medications (Cochrane review). *The Cochrane Library, Issue 2*, Oxford: Update software, 2002.

15. Ley P. Communicating with Patients: Improving Communication, Satisfaction and Compliance. Stanlet Thornes, 1988.

16. Global Alliance for Vaccines and Immunisations http://www.vaccinealliance.org/. 2002.

17. McKeown. The role of Medicine. Dream, mirage or nemesis? Oxford: Blackwell, 1979.

18. Szreter S. The importance of social intervention in Britain's mortality decline c1850-1914: a re-interpretation of the role of public health. *The Society for the social history of Medicine* 1988;2-37.

19. Ramos-Jimenes P, Rodriguez C, Patino O, Lim B. Immunisation in the Philippines. Amsterdam: Het Spinhuis, 1999.

20. Tan M. All in the name of life. *Reproductive health matters* 1995;**6**:29-31.

21. Hispanick J,.Coddington D. The immunisation status of poor children: an analysis of parental altruism and child well-being. *Review of social economy* 2000;**58**:81-107.

22. Riechert T, Sugaya N, Fedson D. The Japanese experience with vaccinating schoolchildren against influenza. *New England Journal of Medicine* 2001;**344**:889-96.

23. Gillon R. Philosophical medical ethics. Chichester: John Wiley and sons, 1986.

24. Pilgrim D,.Rogers A. Mass childhood immunisation - some ethical doubts for primary health care workers. *Nursing Ethics* 1995;**2**:63-70.

25. Kulenkampf M, Schwatzman J, Wilson J. Neurological complications of pertussis inoculation. *Arch Dis Child* 1974;**49**:46-9.

26. Wolfe R,.Sharp L. Anti-vaccinationists past and present. *BMJ* 2002;**325**:430-2.

27. Porter D,.Porter R. The politics of prevention: anti-vaccinationism and public health in nineteenth century England. *Med Hist* 1998;**32**:231-52.

28. Arnold D. Colonizing the body: state medicine and epidemic disease in nineteenth century India. Berkeley: University of California Press, 1993.

29. Sköld P. From inoculation to vaccination: smallpox in Sweden in the eighteenth and nineteenth centuries. *Population studies* 1996;**50**:247-62.

30. Greenough P. Intimidation, coercion and resistance in the final stages of the South Asian smallpox eradication campaign, 1973-1975. *Soc.Sci.Med.* 1995;**41**:633-45.

31. Egers I,.Streefland P. De ontwikkeling van de vaccinatiepraktijk in Nederland (How vaccination practice developed in the Netherlands). *Tijdschrift voor Social Gezondheidszorg* 1997;**75**:28-37.

32. Plotkin S, Plotkin S. A short history of vaccination. In Plotkin S, Orenstein W, eds. *Vaccines*, Philadelphia: Saunders, 1999.

33. New S,.Senior M. "I don't believe in needles": qualitative aspects of a study into the uptake of infant immunisation in two English Health Authorities. *Soc.Sci.Med.* 1991;**33**:509-18.

34. Rogers A, Pilgrim D, Gust I, Stone D, Menzel P. The pros and cons of immunisation. *Health Care Analysis* 1995;**3**:99-115.

35. Sporton R,.Francis F. Choosing not to immunise: are parents making informed decisions? *Family Practice* 2001;**18**:181-8.

36. Bond L, Nolan T, Pattison P, Carlin J. Vaccine preventable diseases and immunisation: a qualitative study of mother's

perceptions of severity, susceptibility, benefits and barriers. *Australian and New Zealand Journal of Public Health* 1998;**22(4)**:441-6.

37.   Marshall S,.Swerissen H. A qualitative analysis of parental decision making for childhood immunisation. *Australian and New Zealand Journal of Public Health* 1999;**23(5)**:543-5.

38.   Evans M, Stoddart H, Freeman E, Grizzell M, Mullen R. Parents' perspectives on the MMR immunisation: a focus group study. *BJGP* 2001;**51**:904-10.

39.   Heggenhougen H, Clements C. Acceptability of Childhood Immunisation: Social Science perspectives. London Publication 14: London School of tropical medicine and hygiene. Evaluation and planning centre for health care, 1987.

40.   Pilsbury B. Immunisation: the behavioural issues. Washington: USAID, 1990.

41.   Markland R,.Durand D. An investigation into socio-psychological factors affecting infant immunisation. *Am J Public Health* 1976;**66**:170.

42.   Strobino D, Keane V, Holt E, Hughart N, Guyer B. Parental attitudes do not explain underimmunisation. *Pediatrics* 1996;1076-83.

43.   Lack of evidence that hepatitis B causes multiple sclerosis. *Weekly epidemiological record* 1997;**72**:149-56.

44.   Simpson N, Lenton S, Randall R. Parental refusal to have children immunised: extent and reasons. *BMJ* 1995;**310**:225-7.

45.   Lack of evidence that hepatitis B causes multiple sclerosis. *Weekly epidemiological record* 1997;**72**:149-56.

46. Lack of evidence that hepatitis B causes multiple sclerosis. *Weekly epidemiological record* 1997;**72**:149-56.

47. Streefland P, Choudhury A, Ramos-Jimenes P. Patterns of vaccination acceptance. *Social Science and Medicine* 1999;**49**:1705-16.

48. Gill E, Sutton S. Immunisation uptake: the role of parental attitudes. In Hey V, ed. *Immunisation research: a summary volume*, London: Health Education Authority, 1998.

49. Rogers A, Pilgrim D. Rational non-compliance with childhood immunisation: personal accounts of parents and primary health care professionals. *Uptake of immunisation: Issues for health educators*, pp 1-67. London: Health Education Authority, 1994.

50. Gust I. The importance of immunisation. *Health Care Analysis* 1995;**3**:107-11.

51. Meszaros J, Asch D, Baron J. Cognitive processes and the decisions of some parents to forgo pertussis vaccination for their children. *Clin Epidemiol* 1996;**49(6)**:697-703.

52. The social science and immunisation research project. *Weekly epidemiological record* 1998;**72**:285-8.

53. Social science and immunisation project website http://www.who.int/vaccines-diseases/Social_Science/socialscience2.shtml. 2002.

54. Streefland P. Enhancing coverage and sustainability of vaccination programs: an explanatory framework with special reference to India. *Social Science and Medicine* 1995;**41**:647-56.

55. Schmidt K,.Ernst E. Survey shows that some homeopaths and chiropractors advise against MMR (letter). *BMJ* 2002;**325**:597.

56. Duffell E. Attitudes of parents towards measles and immunisation following a measles outbreak in an anthroposophical community. *J Epidemiol Community Health* 2001;**55(9)**:685-6.

57. Leask J,.Chapman S. "An attempt to swindle nature": press anti-immunisation reportage 1993-7. *Australian and New Zealand Journal of Public Health* 1998;**22**:17-26.

58. Clements, C. To what extent are vaccine adverse effects a deterrent to immunisation? 1998. Geneva, WHO. Meeting of the scientific advisory group of experts, Global programme for vaccines and immunisation.

59. Justice awareness and basic support. http://www.jabs.org.uk/. 2002.

60. McTaggart L. The vaccination bible. London: WDDTY, 2000.

61. Janz N,.Becker M. The health belief model: a decade later. *Health Educ Q* 1984;**11**:1-47.

62. Rogers R. Cognitive and psychological processes in fear appeals and attitude change: a revised theory of protection motivation. *Social psycho-physiology: a source book*, pp 153-76. New York: Guilford press, 1983.

63. Giddens A. Sociology. Cambridge: Polity Press, 1997.

64. Tajfel H. Differentiation between social groups: Studies in the social psychology of intergroup relations. London: Academic Press, 1978.

65. Middleton E,.Baker D. Trends in the social distribution of MMR coverage in England (1991-2001). *BMJ* 2003;in press.

66. Giddens A. The consequences of modernity. Cambridge: Polity Press, 1991.

67. Giuffrida A, Gosden T, Forland F, Kristiansen I, Sergison M, Leese B *et al.* Target payments in primary care: effects on professional practice and health care outcomes (Cochrane review). *The Cochrane Library, Issue 1*, Oxford: Update software, 2001.

68. Kassianos G. Boosting influenza immunisation for the over 65s. *BJGP* 2002;**52**:710-1.

69. Szilagyi P, Vann J, Bordley C, Chelminski A, Kraus R, Margolis P *et al.* Interventions aimed at improving immunisation rates (Cochrane review). *The Cochrane Library, Issue 4*, Oxford: Update Software, 2002.

70. Stone E, Morton S, Hulscher M, Maglione M, Roth E, Grimshaw J *et al.* Interventions that increase use of adult immunisation and cancer screening services: a meta-analysis. *Ann Intern Med* 2002;**136**:651.

71. Donovan J, Mills N, Smith M, Brindle L, Jacoby A, Peters T *et al.* Quality improvement report: Improving design and conduct of randomised trials by embedding them in qualitative research: ProtecT (prostate testing for cancer and treatment) study. *BMJ* 2002;**325**:766-70.

72. Holm S. Goodbye to simple solutions: the second phase of priority setting. *BMJ* 1998;**317**:1000-2.

73.   Vernon J. The limitations of natural science as applied to medicine. *BJGP* 2002;**52**:870-1.

74.   Bakhtin M. Problems in Dostoyevsky's poetics. Minneapolis: University of Minnesota Press, 1997.

75.   Muir Gray J. Evidence-based healthcare. Churchill Livingstone: New York, 1997.

76.   Sackett D, Strauss S, Richardson S, Rosenberg W, Haynes R. Evidence-based medicine. Edinburgh: Churchill Livingstone, 2000.

77.   Report of the CFS/ME Working Group http://www.doh.gov.uk/cmo/cfsmereport/index.htm. DoH . 2002.

78.   Chapman J. Systems failure: why governments must learn to think differently. London: Desmos, 2002.

79.   Chapman J. A systems perspective on computing in the NHS. *Informatics in primary care* 2002;**10**:199.

80.   Health promotion England's Immunisation Programme http://www.hpe.org.uk/immun.htm. 2002.

81.   MMR - The big questions, a Q & A session for health professionals. 2001. Health promotion England.

82.   MMR - What parents want to know. 2001. Health promotion England.

83.   Health promotion video for MMR http://www.immunisation.org.uk/immresour.html#video. 2002.

84. Health promotion England's Immunisation Programme
     http://www.hpe.org.uk/immun.htm. 2002.

85. DoH. Update on immunisation issues
     http://www.doh.gov.uk/cmo/letters/cmo0204.htm. DoH.
     2002.

86. Nichter M. Vaccinations in the third world: a consideration
     of community demand. *Social Science and Medicine*
     1995;**41**:617-33.

The next article is a summary, never published, of my dissertation for the MSc in General Practice. It was this dissertation which changed my view of human nature. For if altruistic behaviour provides an insoluble dilemma in a rational individualistic framework, the dilemma disappears if we consider people as primarily social beings. The original started with the Herbert poem quoted above in "What is man?" The external examiner told me off. There was a word limit on the project. "If you had not used words on the poem, you would have had more for the footnotes," she said. I could tell there would be no meeting of minds.

Beyond Altruism, A Qualitative Interview Study of Non-family Carers

Abstract
The study asked, "Why do some people choose to care for others to whom they are not tied by duty or financial interest? Can anything be learnt from studying this group about altruism or about carers in general?" The study involved semi-structured interviews with thirty participants recruited mostly in general practice. Many of those cared for were elderly. The analysis indicated that the carers conceived themselves as friends, neighbours or adopted family, rather than as carers. There is typically a relationship of many decades before the need for care becomes apparent and they think about the maintenance of the relationship in terms of duty and love. There are themes about social factors and the social context of care. Care is usually more trouble free if the carer perceives that she is the only person available.

Introduction

The concept of altruism

This project seeks to think about altruism. Its focus is on the general question, "Why should people care for one another?" Some practical suggestions about carers and the ageing population will be considered. The emphasis, however, will be on the question of altruism in an extreme population: non-family carers. These people are spending their time looking after other people, and yet not for reasons of family obligation or for money. Why are they performing altruistic actions?

One possible answer would be that non-family carers possess altruistic motives. Altruism was a word introduced by Comte (Comte 1830) in opposition to egoism. A standard contemporary definition in social psychology would be "helpful acts carried out in the absence of obvious tangible rewards" (Schroeder et al. 1995).

There are traditionally two different motivations for altruism, love and duty, and they are reviewed by Mansbridge (Mansbridge 1990). Love is doing and seeing for the benefit of the other (making the other's good your own), and duty is behaving to the other following some internalised and shared norm. That is, duty can be a principle of beneficence or reciprocity but is to be opposed to rational self-interest.

The model of the person dominant in the economic sciences today can be described as follows. A person is seen as a rational individual. He chooses his actions by deciding what is best for him from his individual point of view. Society is seen simply as an aggregation of pre-existing individuals.

Such a view of human nature inevitably raises the altruism question; "If a person is, by definition, purely self-interested, why should a person care for, or act in the interest of, another person?" This question has accumulated a large literature which has been extensively reviewed (Oliner & Oliner 1988), (Batson 1991) and (Schroeder, Penner, Dovidio, & Piliavin 1995).

However, a view of the person different from the "rational actor" view is possible. The relationship between an individual person and society is more complex than this simple model would have us believe. Indeed, the relationship between the individual and society has been different at different times and in different cultures. Some goods, such as language or money are irreducibly social (Taylor

1989). If we view society as primary then it is the social norms of that society that constitute a person. Self-interest, altruism and reciprocity would themselves all be simply social norms.

This is how sociologists such as Bulmer have seen altruism and reciprocity (Bulmer 1986). He would see both as an exchange of gifts. Under the norm of reciprocity, the gifts exchanged are similar (e.g. friendship for friendship). Under the norm of altruism, the gifts exchanged are different (e.g. care for gratitude).

The classic English sociological text about altruism is Titmuss's study of blood donors, "The gift relationship" (Titmuss 1970). He is keen to point out the wider benefits or "externalities" that are sometimes missed by a narrow economic analysis. In particular he feels that "opportunities to give" are something that should be actively fostered by social policy as they lead to social cohesion and diminish the sense of individual alienation. He reviews the work of anthropologists such as Mauss (Mauss 1954) and Lévi-Strauss (Lévi-Strauss 1955) who have examined the gift relationship in primitive societies. He concludes that such non-economic gifts, made primarily to strengthen social bonds and forge social cohesion, are also important in modern Western societies. His work is very much in line with this study, both in its stress on the importance and relative frequency of altruistic behaviour and in its criticism of a narrowly economic view of persons.

Another classic author is Janet Finch who wrote and researched the question of family obligations for two decades (Finch 1989) (Finch & Mason 1997). She is strong on the analysis of duty in its many contexts, economic and social. She examines the process of negotiation by which decisions are made in a specific case. She is, however, scathing about altruism, calling it "a concept which legitimises the sacrifice of women." She does not mention the word "love" in the book, though some mention is made of emotion. Yet interviews with carers (Qureshi & Walker 1989) and altruists (such as this study) have consistently found that, asked about their motivation, respondents mention both love and duty.

Review of the literature on carers

The General Household Surveys for 1985, 1990, and 1995 and 2000 have given consistent answers as to the number of non-family carers (Rowlands & Parker 1998), ((Maher & Green 2002) table 3.6). On each occasion 3 per cent of adults have said that they look after a friend or neighbour, making them about 18 per cent of all carers. This works out at about 1.0 million non-family carers in the UK. Of these, 204,000 non-family carers, or 0.6 per cent of the adult population work for greater than 20 hours per week (Rowlands & Parker 1998), ((Maher & Green 2002) table 4.6). Work on the number of non-kin or non-family carers has been reviewed (Nocon & Pearson 2000).

There have been two large-scale semi-structured interview studies of family carers in the UK (Qureshi & Walker 1989) and (Twigg & Atkin 1994). They consider "non-kin" carers as having "a limited role to play". However the definition of kin relationships is itself partially socially defined (Strathern 1992). The present study found, without difficulty, a number of carers who explained their actions on the basis of kin ties, "I look after her because she is like a mum to me". These were kin ties which were purely socially defined and which had no biological content.

This strand of research has been summarised as showing that "care takes place within an existing relationship" which, according to "Caring for carers" (DoH (Department of Health) 1999), "is characterised by bonds of obligation, affection, and reciprocity". The context of care is an existing relationship. Would this also apply to non-family carers? Both studies, (Qureshi & Walker 1989) and (Twigg & Atkin 1994), generated a typology of carer motivation; normative factors (within the family set-up), affect and reciprocity.

More recent work on carers has moved on from the early focus on the "burden of care". The disability rights movement has emphasised that the goal of the disabled person may not be independence but autonomy (Morris 1998) (Shakespeare 2000). By this is meant that the cared-for person should be in charge of the help that they receive. Finally some writers have based themselves on a feminist ethic of care (Sevenhuijsen 2000) (Lloyd 2003). For them having friends, social connections, or social capital in Putnam's phrase (Putnam 2000), is the most important value of all. As one of them has put it; "In the end, caring relationships are what we all (both carers and service users) need." (Lloyd 2003)

There has been one published qualitative study devoted solely to care provided by friends and neighbours (Nocon & Pearson 2000). That paper, unlike this project, has a focus on policy issues. It has an excellent summary of previous work in this field. It does not consider "quasi-kin" relationships. One big advantage it has over this study was that they were able to interview some of the "cared-for" as well as the carers. On related topics there is some literature on networks of care (Wenger 1994) (Bytheway & Johnson 1998), and case managed volunteers as carers (Qureshi, Challis, & Davies 1989). Research on carers has recently been summarised by Stalker (Stalker 2003) and Stevenson (Stevenson 2003).

Social psychology

Social psychology is probably the discipline that has been most directly interested in caring behaviour (Schroeder, Penner, Dovidio, & Piliavin 1995). The best studied caring behaviour is by-stander intervention. There is a well-known model that describes it (Latané & Darley 1970). One important step of this model is that bystanders are much more likely to help if they perceive that there is "nobody else near". If other people are near "diffusion of social responsibility" occurs, and bystanders are less likely to help.

A qualitative social psychology literature on caring has also developed, chiefly in the USA, (Farran et al. 1991), (Gubrium & Sankar 1994), (Miller et al. 1997). This literature aims to understand "how one's life is altered by becoming and being a caregiver" ((Lyman 1994) p.158.). A study of carers of people with dementia, in the existentialist tradition, described how the carer "creates or discovers meaning" in the act of caring (Farran 1997). Another qualitative study of family carers was carried out in

France (Grand et al. 1999). In this study the following became clear; firstly the caring relationship involves an on-going negotiation between the two parties, not a one-off decision (see also Finch 1989). Secondly where there are several possible carers the negotiation between these possible carers is a major feature and often leads to friction.

As well as these theoretical aspects, there should also be practical benefits from research into non-family carers. The need for more carers is widely felt. Because of shrinking public support for the welfare state, and an ageing population, the government accepts that this need for carers will increase (Pickard et al. 2000). Because of the continuing fragmentation of the extended family there will be increasing scope for "non-family" carers. How can we best recruit and encourage carers? To do this we need to see the world from their point of view and qualitative analysis of carers' interviews enables us to do so. Moreover, some reflections about them, and in particular how they think about caring, should be generalisable to all carers.

Methods

The definition of a non-family carer is the person seen by the person cared-for as their chief or almost chief carer. Exclusions are: first degree relatives, a financial motive known or suspected, or an affective relationship prior to the onset of care.

As far as reflexivity is concerned the interviewer openly identified himself as a general practitioner that is a British family doctor or GP, and dressed as such, with the following effects. Criticism of the health service was restrained or absent. Some respondents may have taken the interview as recognition of their activities and been encouraged in them. A one-hour interview was powerful enough to allow disclosure of one case of childhood physical abuse and one of sexual abuse. One carer clearly expressed extreme anger to the cared-for on tape. Many carers implied that this was the first time they had reflected on their behaviour. Clearly such enforced reflection could alter their behaviour.

Recruitment

Recruitment was a two-stage process. In the first stage a GP or other informant (who had been contacted by the researcher personally) identified a non-family carer, obtained their consent, and passed the name of the non-family carer back to the researcher. The researcher (who is a GP) then contacted the carer directly. Most respondents were recruited via GPs.

Recruitment was in two stages because of the problem of consent. It is also the case that nomination by a trusted person was an essential step in recruitment because very few of the respondents would have identified themselves as carers.

Table 1; Recruitment: the numbers of respondents recruited by source.

Total respondents	Recruited by	Recruited by (detail)	numbers
all = 30	GPs = 23	Of which; self	8
		one partner	3
		Trainers	7; from 6 GPs
		Primary care group	2; from 1 GP
		GP friends	3; one each
	Informants = 5	Mrs. V. (organiser)	2
		Mrs. S. (carer)	2
		Mrs. L. (ex-carer)	1
	churches = 1		1
	District Nurses = 1	Local clinic	1

The semi-structured interview

The semi-structured interview was based on the literature. There were an initial few questions to elicit the basic demographic data. Then there was a section on the onset and continuation of the relationship based on the Latané and Darley model of bystander intervention (Latané & Darley 1970). There is a final section on background and upbringing. Questions based on the Latané and Darley model included; can you tell me something about how you met? How did you first notice the need? Why did you assume personal responsibility? What made you think you could help?

Coding was carried out after all the interviews were finished. The interviews were transcribed. The researcher, in collaboration with Dr Jane Ogden (see acknowledgments), devised the coding scheme, eventually containing 97 separate codes. We performed axial coding (Strauss & Corbin 1998), and then coded the interviews using Atlas.ti.

An attempt was made to assess inter-rater reliability. Four interviews were re-coded by the transcriber. The number of quotations to which she attached exactly the same code as the first coder (the researcher) was 119/172 or 69 per cent. This statistic is called inter-rater reliability ((Miles & Huberman 1984). Miles and Huberman reckon suggest that 70 per cent is average for a first check on inter-rater reliability. Re-coding with a second coder allowed detailed discussion of the codes.

The interviews were analysed following coding in Atlas.ti. For the first few interviews all comments were allocated a code. Thereafter, although the interviews were read line by line, a code was only allocated if a comment appeared not to fit into the existing coding scheme, so that a new code was generated, or the comment was a striking illustration of an existing code. An example of a new code is "care of pets", a frequent code not anticipated in the original scheme. The codes were grouped into themes (axial coding). Coding and analysis did not strictly follow "grounded theory" (Strauss & Corbin 1998) although it was inspired by elements of this method.

Results

There were thirty interviews. Names and some details have been changed to preserve confidentiality.

Quantitative description of the sample

The carers' ages ranged from 30-80 years, with a mean of 60 years. The age of the cared-for ranged from 35-95 years, with a mean of 80 years. Sex of the carer (25 women and 5 men) and cared-for (20 women and 10 men) showed a predominance of women but all permutations of the sexes were included, to ensure a diverse sample. This was possible because more respondents were offered than could be interviewed. The same diversity is found when considering place of residence. Finally, the duration of relationship was strikingly long, running from 1 to 60 years, with a median of 20 years. Within this long relationship it was often difficult to define the moment when caring started but it was typically of many years standing. The caring ranged in intensity from "keeping an eye on" to virtually twenty four hour care of an elderly neighbour dying of motor neurone disease. No attempt was made to estimate the number of hours of care. While the principal disability was old age this included various elements of physical and mental disability. For example, one old lady had severe Alzheimer's whereas another, mentioned above, died of motor neurone disease. There were also examples of the following situations: an alcoholic woman, a homeless man, a single mother and an adult with a congenital mental disability.

Analysis by themes

After analysis of the reasons that the carers chose to care the following themes emerged:

1) the nature of the pre-existing relationship,
2) the identity of the carer,
3) the role of duty and love in the maintenance of the relationship,
4) the social context of the care.

Preliminary note - the use of the word "carer"

The word "carer" is widely used in the literature and in government documents. Yet it was rarely used spontaneously by the respondents. It was only used three times in all and each time with reservations:

> "Yes. But it wasn't a drudge to care for him. It was quite a pleasant feeling I had of myself that I was helping someone, you see." (7)

Here the carer is repudiating the secondary meaning of care as drudge. Or:

> "And I think, to be quite honest, I think I quite like caring for people. I don't think I'd do it otherwise." (28)

Here the carer is underlining the voluntary nature of her care. The carers preferred to use expressions like "help", "put myself out", or "just normal".

The nature of the relationship

Perhaps the key theme to emerge was the carer's concept of the relationship, that is the name which the carer uses to describe their relationship with the cared-for. There are four common concepts of the nature of the relationship: friend, neighbour, adopted family, or cared-for replacing a loved one. It was, for most carers, because they were in a pre-existing relationship that care started. This is known to be the case for family carers (DoH (Department of Health) 1999).

Friendship is the most common description of the relationship (21/30). They have often been friends for decades before one friend falls ill. They see friendship as a mutual relationship voluntarily entered into. Friends choose each other, though this may be by instinct rather than a conscious choice. Friendship implies reciprocity:

> "And it seems to be a two-way thing, helping each other. So if we're away on holiday she'll come in and water the plants. And gardening has been something that has made

the friendship develop because we'll ask her advice over it. So that has helped." (13)

The implication here appears to be that friendship requires more reciprocity and equity than does "being a neighbour". The norm of equity requires that both friends put something into the friendship. The friendship may originate over a cup of tea, a business deal, or mutual friends, but it becomes "friendship that lasts". That is, friendship that lasts when one of the friends falls ill.

> "C: I suppose the friendship was there. And I can't just drop a friend when they need help, in my opinion." (29)

The norm of equity has to be maintained in this now changed friendship. It may be maintained by delayed reciprocity, by other forms of help or by the expression of gratitude.

The term "adopted family" was applied in twelve cases. This generally is taken to mean a strong commitment and implies that the care will last until death. In the following extract the carer explains how and when she made an explicit commitment to her "adopted mum":

"I: Did you ever think there was going to be an end to the relationship?

> C: No, no. Once I've made a commitment it's not fair to, is it? Because they rely on you and if there is nobody else then it's important that they know that somebody's always there for them.
>
> I: Did you explicitly tell her that?
>
> C: Yes. Yes.
>
> I: In what way?
>
> C: I think probably when she had the cancer of the tongue." (9)

While there were four who were seen as "second mum", every possible role in a family was allocated to the cared-for.

If the relationship is seen as that of <u>neighbours</u> this always implies a degree of distance:

> "We've always been good neighbours, never been in and out of each other's houses, but we've always been good neighbours." (4)

And it implies of a neighbourhood, a degree of privacy:

> "Because we are of a helpful neighbourhood here inasmuch as we have very good neighbours and everybody is interested in everybody – not in an interfering way." (12)

Being a neighbour is less a relationship of choice than is being a friend. It does not imply liking, and friendship may be denied: The strength of neighbourly feeling may be more dependent on social than personal factors, as the following perceptive comment implies:

> "We live in an area here, or with people here, which is a bit of a caring part. But I think one of the main reasons for that is the fact that we live in cul-de-sac. ... You get to know the people better and you get a feeling of responsibility towards each other. ..." (12)

Self-concept as neighbour, in contrast to friend and adopted family, implies moving can interrupt the commitment, as was the case in two respondents.

Finally, the relationship might be conceived of as <u>the cared-for person replacing a loved one</u>. In many cases this was no more than a background hint, but twice it was completely explicit:

> "Yes, I think of her as an adopted mother because my mother died four years ago, nearly five years ago, and I suppose why I help [her] was because my mother lived in Sheffield and I was still working. And although we used to go up there about every ten or twelve weeks, and my brother lives up there, I felt that I didn't do as much for her as I would have liked to. So I felt that this was probably, I was helping [her] because I couldn't help mum." (9)

This was also the case of a schoolteacher who took over the care of an old man from her best friend who was dying of cancer.

Summary of nature of the relationship

The importance of the concept of the relationship which the carers have is that it alters the attributions they can make and with the different relationships come different public social duties. If you choose a certain relationship then you choose the norms and duties that go with it. If the nature of the relationship with someone you care for is "like mother" it will involve more onerous responsibilities than "like neighbour". To be specific when the nature was "adopted family" the commitment was understood to be until death; whereas the commitment "like neighbour" is understood to terminate when one party moves. The social duties of a friend are intermediate, and on this relationship the norm of equity weighs more heavily.

The identity of the carer

The phrase "the carer's identity" means how they see themselves. They may see themselves as carers, or as professional carers, or their identity might be based on their religion. Those who have an identity as carers are those who say their purpose, or meaning in life, is in caring relationships. For these people their personal identity was a strong reason for continuing to be carers, and it gave meaning to their lives (Farran, Keane-Hagerty, Salloway, Kupferer, & Wilken 1991). For most people, however, it was the continuing relationship, not their identity that was important.

Five respondents had an identity as a <u>professional carer</u>. They were retired members of the caring professions (four nurses, one social worker). For them it seemed clear that their professional identity had a role in their present behaviour. It might be perceived as socially expected:

> "I'm a nurse; I've lived here most of my life. Everybody knows that. If I had an elderly lady living next door who couldn't cope, and I lived next door, and everybody said, well, "Why didn't she do something?"" (24)

Or the act of caring might restore an identity threatened by retirement. In the following quotation, a retired nurse, who has moved into a block of retirement flats, is asked what the cared-for has done for her:

> "Well, really she's done nothing for me apart from the fact that I feel myself to be useful once again, which is very important." (18)

To have or to choose an identity is to choose certain extra social norms to follow over and above those normal for all members of that society. It is by enacting those norms that the identity is both internally confirmed and externally displayed.

For others, their identity as a <u>carer</u> was the purpose or meaning of their life. Both those brought up as carers, and those who become carers by adult choice, may forge themselves an identity as carers. For example, one carer, who was in the building trade, had devoted himself to looking after his male partner until his partner died of AIDS. This experience, (which occurred prior to the non-family caring relationship about which he was interviewed for this project), changed him:

> C "It's my vocation in life, if you like, is to go out and look after somebody. Whether you get paid for it or whether you don't – that's immaterial. If you get paid for it, it's secondary.

> I: That would be nice, but it is secondary.

> C: Yes.

> I: When did it become clear to you that that was your vocation in life?

> C: When I looked after [my partner]." (21)

For as the poet Gerald Manley Hopkins wrote:

> "This seeing the sick endears them to us, us too it endears."

How we choose to understand our caring depends on our identity and the nature of the relationship, but acts of caring will in turn alter how we see ourselves.

Could identity as a carer be based on religion? This turned out to be a rarely mentioned theme. Perhaps because North Essex is predominantly white the only religion mentioned by the respondents was Christianity. Identity as a Christian was only mentioned as cause of caring behaviour four times:

> "I'm a Christian – I believe that we are here to help other people. I mean, what is your purpose in life – everybody's purpose is different – I would not be happy with myself if I didn't do what I considered to be my best." (26)

Others may not have mentioned it; one (although a Christian) explicitly denied it:

> "Well, we don't do it because we think it's our Christian duty, we feel it's a natural thing to do." (12)

The maintenance of the relationship (love or duty)

Maintenance of the relationship depends on the altruistic motives of the carer. As discussed in the introduction, altruistic motivations can be classified as duty or love.

Conformity to social norms (duty, conscience).

Conformity to social norms is doing one's duty. If the norms are internalised it can be seen as obeying one's conscience. Many of the respondents' comments could be analysed under the norms of reciprocity, equity, and social responsibility.

Reciprocity was not perceived as part of human nature, as in the "rational actor" view of the person. Rather reciprocity was viewed as a social norm, or duty:

> "She's done a lot for me, so I feel it's my duty to look after to her." (14)

This is the norm of specific reciprocity which is specific to a particular relationship. But there is also a norm of general reciprocity. This is the belief that if you help one person you will be helped by a quite different person later on. If you followed the norm of general reciprocity it appeared to give you an expectation, however illusory, that you yourself would be helped when you needed it:

> "I don't think you lose anything by helping people.
> Because I know that people would always help me. I've
> always got that feeling that they would help me." (20)

The norm of equity implies the need for balance in a relationship. This norm is threatened when one person begins to need care. For the care to proceed this balance must therefore be redressed. This need for balance is primarily met by the cared-for expressing gratitude, but also by other sorts of help given by the cared-for. There also seemed to be a sense in which the cared-for had to show that they were a deserving person in terms of their qualities or the help they had previously given.

The expression of gratitude was a marked feature of almost all accounts. For example:

> "I: Is she grateful, or resentful, or...?
>
> C: No, grateful. Oh, extremely grateful. Never resentful, never resentful.
>
> I: When she expresses her gratitude, she says, makes it clear that she's...?
>
> C: Oh absolutely, yes. We have to have a hug a day." (9)

If gratitude was not expressed, the carer had to assume it was there nevertheless:

> "I think in her way she's grateful. But she doesn't show it.
> But she is. I'm sure she is. She doesn't actually show it.
> But that's just how she is. That's the type of person she is."
> (19)

The expression of gratitude restores the norm of equity. In voluntary relationships like these it is essential; unless the carer can in some way attribute gratitude to the cared-for, the relationship will come to an end.

The carer undertakes to help, at least in part, because he imputes "deserving" qualities to the person he is helping. A particular emphasis was made on the cared-for being a helper herself in the days when she was able:

> "She is somebody quite like myself. She would do anything for anybody." (5)

There are many mentions of current practical help from the cared-for. Most often mentioned are the pleasures of friendship: emotional support, interesting conversation, stories, and the sheer joy of knowing people. There could be help with gardening, business, or hobbies.

Another important social norm is that of <u>social responsibility or altruism</u>. As Schroeder puts it; "According to this social norm, people are expected to help others who are dependent on them" ((Schroeder, Penner, Dovidio, & Piliavin 1995) p.87). As one respondent put it:

> "She was a person that needed help and if I could help her, I would. That was it. I just got on with it." (5)

Love as a motive for caring

Love is well defined by the following quotation from Mansbridge; "By love I mean making another's goods [and perspective] my own," ((Mansbridge 1990) p.135.)

Love often starts with emotional empathy, that is; a feeling for somebody in distress:

> "Yes. My heart broke for her at the time." (3)

Rather notoriously, emotional empathy does not necessarily lead to action.

So that emotional empathy needs to be followed by cognitive empathy; that is seeing life from another's perspective:

> "I mean, I put myself in her place. And I thought: I know what I would be like." (27)

Typically, the carers perceived that the people they were helping wanted personal rather than impersonal care. Cognitive empathy then needs to be followed by action.

Acting from another's perspective is more costly than "just doing the job"; it takes time and imagination:

> "I don't think an old person wants you to go in and give their breakfast and walk out, they don't want that." (1)

It is also costly when the relationship ends and could lead to a strong sense of bereavement.

The social context of care

Reasons for caring include the social context of care, in particular negotiations with other potential providers. Three themes emerged concerning the social context of care. These were the theme of "nobody else near", and the themes of negotiation with other relatives (Finch 1989), and with statutory institutions.

The theme of "nobody else near" was already identified by Grand (Grand, Grand-Filaire, Bocquet, & Clement 1999). It is easier to commit oneself to the burden of care if one perceives that nobody else is available. This is analogous to the concept in social psychology of "diffusion of social responsibility". The respondents often mentioned this, and there were only two counter-examples. The situation was expressed by one of them as follows:

> "Maybe most people think: someone else will do it.
> Someone else will do it – well let's not bother, someone

else will do it. But I think if that person knows that there really isn't anybody else that will do it, I think most people would if there was really no alternative." (17)

The theme of <u>negotiation with family</u> was very frequent. The family was generally kept informed of the situation. Mostly they were too far away, or too committed in other ways to be realistic alternative providers of care. Hence the relations were harmonious and did not interfere with the carer's perception that there was "nobody else near", or lead to diffusion of responsibility. There was an especially close liaison on financial matters. The only disagreement with a relative occurred about money:

> "No, she was rude to me, in a way she was rude – I'd got her mother's pension for her and I'd paid her electric bill for her and I said, would you like the money? And she said, "Yes I would!" She said, "I'll take it now!" As though I was going to take it from her." (29)

Often there was close communication in networks of carers. Organised voluntary care only featured in one account and that in a peripheral role.

The theme of <u>negotiation with institutions, social and health services</u> was less frequent. Some contact with social services had probably occurred in most cases, especially with the occupational therapy department and meals on wheels. However, the general perception was that further care was either unavailable, or unacceptable to the cared-for. In such cases there was clearly no scope for conflict. Two middle-class carers reported successful negotiations with social services leading to extensive provision of services.

Two other carers had less success. One was a neighbour on a council housing estate. She tried to leave messages for the carers, but was rebuffed:

> "Going back to a few months ago when I was going round there and finding her wet, I used to leave notes on bits of paper for the carers to say, please could you take her to the

toilet when you come in of an evening. And I got a note left for me telling me basically I wasn't to tell the carers what to do." (8)

Another neighbour clearly felt coerced into providing temporary care:

"The first two weeks social services didn't send anybody in. And the social worker said, couldn't [the neighbour] do it? Well it was that or her not coming home [from hospital]." (25)

Nor did the care package arrive smoothly after two weeks but only after what the carer felt was "a nightmare" of delayed or broken promises.

Discussion

Practical issues

This is the second study to focus solely on non-family carers. In contrast to the first study (Nocon & Pearson 2000) recruitment was via primary care. Nocon and Pearson's respondents were largely recruited through voluntary agencies. The rich description given in their study is, however, recognisably similar to the situation here. This study has confirmed the significance of the care given by non-family carers. The significance of the care has been defined from the perspective of the person cared-for, rather than from a policy perspective. Qureshi (Qureshi & Walker 1989) long ago showed that, where family are available, they will generally provide the care. Hence most of the cared-for, who have non-family carers, are isolated from their families. The care provided by non-family carers is highly significant to them and may be their chief or only contact with the outside world.

Are there any differences between family and non-family carers? The typology of care is strikingly similar in both cases. This is described in "Caring for carers" as; "obligation, affection, and reciprocity" (DoH (Department of Health) 1999).However there is less obvious reciprocity in the case of non-family carers. They are also less likely to feel trapped as it is a voluntary relationship which they can choose to terminate without incurring social disapproval. Perception of need generally occurs through pre-existing relationships, as is the case for family carers (Qureshi & Walker 1989). This is quite different from perception of need in bystander intervention (Latané & Darley 1970). Some, but not all carers, have an identity as a carer or professional carer. While some report socialisation into caring as children, others were socialised as young adults. Those who were socialised as adults tended to form "ideal" relationships to replace those with their natural parents whose values they no longer shared.

Care can provide meaning to some carers (Farran 1997), but not all the non-family carers. It is those carers with an identity as a carer, or as a professional carer, for whom caring provides meaning. In most cases there is a strong pre-existing relationship and the meaning comes from that relationship.

The social setting may be important, especially the perception that "there is no-one else near". In this project the concept of "diffusion of social responsibility" from the social psychology literature has been generalised. It has been applied to interactions, not only with other potential carers, but also with institutions like social services. It helps to explain why the entry of social services offering help can lead to conflict. This conflict has been noted by others, though different explanations are offered. For example Nocon suggested that "the resentment that some express about arrangements indicates that they feel they have been pulled across a normative boundary" (Nocon & Pearson 2000). Twigg long ago described the practice "in some areas" of seeing the availability of informal care as a reason for not providing formal services (Twigg & Atkin 1994).

Social services have traditionally seen themselves as providers of care and assessors of need, with the carers seen as a passive resource (see table 2, line 1 below). One first step, in increasing carer involvement, described as long ago as 1989, is to see carers as co-workers or co-clients (see table 2, line 2 below) (Twigg 1989), (Twigg & Atkin 1994). This is the idea behind the assessment of carers by social services as envisaged by the Carers and Disabled Children's Act (2000). A further step is to involve carers as partners. This is the rhetoric of "Caring for Carers" (DoH (Department of Health) 1999) and the Griffith report (Griffith 1988), but observational studies have shown how difficult it can be to achieve this change in culture (see table 2, line 3 below) (Goss & Miller 1995). A final step would be to see part of the role of social services as fostering communities and strengthening social bonds, as in Professor Putnam's seminal American book "Bowling alone" (Putnam 2000) or the later work of the Oliners (Oliner & Oliner 1995) (see table 2, line 4 below). This last perspective is one of the communitarian policies, advocated by these authors, which would strengthen social bonds and reduce alienation in society. It is a perspective close to that of the feminist ethics of care (Lloyd 2003), Shakespeare's interdependence (Shakespeare 2000), or Williams's "new political ethic of care" which would promote care as "a social process engendering important elements of citizenship." ((Williams 2001) p.477.)

Table 2; A hierarchy of social service involvement with carers

1	*Carers as a resource; (still the usual situation today).*
2	Carers as co-workers or co-clients; (Twigg & Atkin 1994).
3	Carers (and cared for) as partners in planning services; (Goss & Miller 1995).
4	Carers (and cared for) as partners in "increasing social capital"; (Putnam 2000).

A further implication for social services is that, if the carers use the language of love and duty and not that of rational choice, then it follows that those that wish to engage with them should do so using the same language. This means that documents written for carers should not be afraid to talk of duty and love, though clearly this language should not be used as an excuse to exploit carers. Again, as has been noted before, if "carers" do not recognise the word "carer" as applying to them, it cannot be used in literature aimed at them (Stalker 2004).

Methodological limitations

While the method used in this study is good at allowing us to see the world from the carers' perspective, it has considerable limitations. It cannot look directly at learning and socialisation. It cannot examine arousal and emotion which are often seen as the motors of care. These might be better investigated in the social psychology laboratory (Batson 1991). Because they were not interviewed, it tells us nothing about the relationship from the point of view of the cared-for. It tells us little about the quality of the help; enough perhaps to begin to research it, but not enough to recommend it as a source of care at present.

Theoretical implications

By seeing carers as partially socially constituted (MacIntyre 1985) (Vernon 2003) we can get beyond the dichotomy between altruism and egoism. The carers interviewed spoke primarily the language of social norms. The language of rational choice hardly occurs. Hence it would be fair to say that the carers see themselves as socially constituted rather than as rational actors. If the carers see altruism as a social norm the problem of altruism does not arise. This is because the problem of altruism only arises if we see the person as a purely rational actor.

The position that human nature is partially socially constituted is explicitly post-modern in suggesting that two contrasting approaches, social norms and rational choice, can be used simultaneously to grasp parts of the truth.

References

Batson, C. 1991, *The altruism question: towards a social psychological answer* Lawrence Erlbaum Associates, Inc., New Jersey.

Bulmer, M. 1986, *Neighbours: the works of Philip Abrams* Cambridge University Press, Cambridge.

Bytheway, B. & Johnson, J. 1998, "The social construction of carers," in *The social construction of care*, A. Symonds & A. Kelly, eds., Macmillan, Basingstoke.

Comte, A. 1830, *Cours de philosophie positive* Bachelier, Paris.

DoH (Department of Health) 1999, *Caring about carers: a national strategy for carers* Department of Health, London.

Farran, C. 1997, "Theoretical perspectives concerning positive aspects of caring for elderly persons with dementia: stress/adaptation and existentialism.", *Gerontologist*, vol. 37, no. 2, pp. 250-255.

Farran, C., Keane-Hagerty, E., Salloway, S., Kupferer, S., & Wilken, C. 1991, "Finding meaning: an alternative paradigm for Alzheimer's disease family caregivers.", *Gerontologist*, vol. 31, pp. 483-489.

Finch, J. 1989, *Family obligations and social change* Polity Press, Cambridge.

Finch, J. & Mason, J. 1997, "Filial obligations and kin support for elderly people," J. Bornat, ed., Open University, Basingstoke.

Goss, S. & Miller, C. 1995, *From margin to mainstream; developing user- and carer-centred community care* Joseph Rowntree Foundation, York.

Grand, A., Grand-Filaire, A., Bocquet, H., & Clement, S. 1999, "Care giver stress: a failed negotiation? A qualitative study in South-West France.", *Int'l.J.Aging and Human Development*, vol. 49, no. 3, pp. 179-195.

Griffith, R. 1988, *Community care; an agenda for action* DHSS, HMSO, London.

Gubrium, J. & Sankar, J. 1994, *Qualitative methods in ageing research* Sage, Thousand Oaks.

Latané, B. & Darley, J. 1970, *The unresponsive bystander; Why doesn't he help?* Appleton-Century-Crofts, New-York.

Lévi-Strauss, C. 1955, *Tristes Tropiques* Librairie Plon, Paris.

Lloyd, L. 2003, "Caring relationships: beyond "carers" and "service users"," in *Reconceptualising work with "carers"*, pp. 37-55.

Lyman, K. 1994, "Field work in groups and institutions," in *Qualitative methods in aging research*, J. Gubrium & J. Sankar, eds., Sage, Thousand Oaks.

MacIntyre, A. 1985, *After Virtue*, 2nd edn, Duckworth, London.

Maher, J. & Green, H. 2002, *Carers 2000: results from the carers' module of the General Household Survey 2000* Stationery Office, London.

Mansbridge, J. 1990, "On the relation of altruism and self-interest," in *Beyond self-interest*, Mansbridge J.J., ed., University of Chicago Press, Chicago, pp. 133-146.

Mauss, M. 1954, *The Gift* Free Press, New York.

Miles, M. & Huberman, M. 1984, *Qualitative data analysis* Sage Publications, Beverley Hills.

Miller, B., Powell Lawton, M., Kramer, B., Beach, D., & Farran, C. 1997, "Symposium: Positive aspects of caregiving.", *Gerontologist*, vol. 37, no. 2, pp. 216-257.

Morris, J. 1998, "Creating a space for absent voices: disabled women's experiences of receiving assistance with daily living activities," in *Understanding health and social care: an introductory reader*, M. M. Allott, ed., Sage, London.

Nocon, A. & Pearson, M. 2000, "The role of friends and neighbours in providing support for older people", *Ageing and Society*, vol. 8, no. 30, pp. 341-367.

Oliner, P. & Oliner, S. 1995, *Toward a caring society: Ideas into action* Praeger Publishers/Greenwood Publishing Group, Inc., Westport, CT, USA.

Oliner, S. & Oliner, P. 1988, *The altruistic personality: Rescuers of Jews in Nazi Europe* The Free Press, New York.

Pickard, L., Wittenberg, R., Comas-Herrera, A., Davies, B., & Darton, R. 2000, "Relying on informal care in the new century? Informal care for elderly people in England to 2031", *Ageing and Society*, vol. 29, pp. 745-772.

Putnam, R. 2000, *Bowling alone* Simon and Schuster, New York.

Qureshi, H., Challis, D., & Davies, B. 1989, *Helpers in case-managed community care* Gower, Aldershot.

Qureshi, H. & Walker, A. 1989, *The caring relationship: elderly people and their families* Macmillan education, Basingstoke.

Rowlands, O. & Parker, G. 1998, *Informal carers: an independent study carried out by the Office for National Statistics on behalf of the Department of Health as part of the 1995 General Household Survey* The Stationery Office, London.

Schroeder, J., Penner, L., Dovidio, J., & Piliavin, J. 1995, *The Psychology of helping and altruism: problems and puzzles* McGraw-Hill, New York.

Sevenhuijsen, S. 2000, "Caring in the third way: the relation between obligation responsibility and care in Third Way discourse", *Critical social policy*, vol. 20, no. 1, pp. 5-37.

Shakespeare, T. 2000, "The social relations of care," in *Rethinking social policy*, G. Lewis, S. Gerwitz, & J. Clarke, eds., Open University Press, Bucks.

Stalker, K. 2003, *Reconceptualising work with "carers"* Jessica Kingsley Publishers, London.

Stalker, K. 2004, "Carers: an overview of concepts developments and debates," in *Reconceptualising work with "carers"*, K. Stalker, ed., Jessica Kingsley Publishers, London, pp. 15-36.

Stevenson, F. 2003, "Community care and informal caring," in *Sociology as applied to medicine*, **5th** edn, G. Scambler, ed., Edinburgh, Saunders, pp. 248-264.

Strathern, M. 1992, *After Nature* Cambridge University Press, Cambridge.

Strauss, A. & Corbin, C. 1998, *Basics of qualitative research: Techniques and procedures for developing grounded theory*, 2nd edn, SAGE publications, Thousand Oaks, California.

Taylor, C. "Irreducibly social goods", Australian National University, Canberra.

Titmuss, R. 1970, *The Gift Relationship: From human blood to Social Policy* George Allen & Unwin, London.

Twigg, J. 1989, "Models of carers: how do social care agencies conceptualise their relationship with informal carers?", *Journal of social policy*, vol. 18, pp. 53-66.

Twigg, J. & Atkin, K. 1994, *Carers perceived; policy and practice in informal care* Open University Press, Buckingham.

Vernon, G. 2003, "What is man?", *BJGP*, vol. 53, pp. 504-505.

Wenger, C. 1994, *Understanding support networks and community care* Avebury, Aldershot.

Williams, F. 2001, "In and beyond New Labour: Towards a new political ethics of care", *Critical social policy*, vol. 21, no. 4, pp. 467-493.

The last of these longer articles appeared in the August 2001 edition of the Catholic Medical Quarterly. The opinions expressed I no longer hold, nevertheless the questions addressed remain topical. Indeed, to my surprise, it continues to be downloaded from the ResearchGate website.

I have changed my mind since writing this piece and no longer see patients seeking an abortion; a notice in the waiting room makes this clear. After writing the piece I came to realise that I was doing this counselling, not because it was any help to the patient, but because I felt pressure from my partners (pressure which they had never expressed) to see patients wanting an abortion.

Can there be a moral dialogue between Doctor and Patient?

Introduction

I want to use the familiar model of a consultation between a British general practitioner and a patient requesting a termination as a model for the wider category of consultations where a moral dialogue might occur. Some general practitioners hold that the foetus is an entity to whom they owe a moral obligation. For such general practitioners the request for a termination poses two moral dilemmas. The dilemma I want to discuss is not that between the rights of the foetus and those of the mother. That dilemma has been well covered from various points of view in the literature on medical ethics (Gillon 1994) and in popular books (Donellan 1997; Lloyd 1996; Wyatt 1998). The dilemma I want to discuss is; "To what extent and in what way should the practitioner engage with the mother in moral dialogue? Can it indeed be done at all?" By moral dialogue I mean a conversation between the two parties, in terms of concepts they share, that helps to form the moral decision of one party. While this dilemma has not been much discussed in England, debate about it has divided the Roman Catholic Church in Germany (The Independent 2000). Moreover, the disability rights lobby has usefully reminded us that the abortion consultation is not purely a private matter, but is one that sends a message to the wider society about how we value disabled people (Shakespeare 1998).

I want to address this question from the perspective of the doctor who feels that his obligation to the foetus is so strong it is not a private matter but rather a universal obligation. By a universal obligation I mean one like the rule "do not kill" which most people feel applies not just to them but to all citizens whatever their other beliefs. Such a doctor feels on the one hand that he should protect the foetus while on the other hand he wishes to respect the autonomy of the mother. This perspective is that of most Roman Catholics, some Protestants, and most Jews and Muslims. Moreover, it is but one of many such dilemmas that arise in our multicultural society in which minority beliefs are often pitted against the quite different norms of wider society.

Historically there are at least three ways that minority groups respond to this challenge: these are mirrored by the range of responses such doctors can give in this situation. Firstly, the group can cut itself off from society into an internal ghetto. This would correspond to the doctor who put a sign in his waiting-room saying he did not see patients for termination. This is the attitude recommended by some Roman Catholic moralists (Finnis & Fisher 1994). Secondly groups can assimilate fully into society, keeping their beliefs, if at all, a private matter. This would correspond to a doctor who behaved as he thought other doctors in the host society behaved, keeping his beliefs for himself. Thirdly the group can engage the host society in a dialogue in various ways. This is the option for the doctor that I want to explore at greater length. I will ask;

1. Is moral dialogue between a doctor and a patient possible in our society?
2. Ought we to engage in it?
3. How can it be done?

The scope of moral obligations

Although I will focus on the dilemma for the doctor I will briefly consider the scope of moral obligations, and whether the foetus is included in them. This is because our attitude to abortion seems to depend principally on this question and much less on which moral theory we follow (Gillon 1986).

Historically over the centuries there has been much fluctuation in opinions about the stage of its development at which the foetus entered the scope of such obligations (Mori 1994). The language used was that of ensoulment; once the foetus had a soul we had obligations to it. Such a debate has not yet died in Roman Catholicism (Mon 1994).

The argument from uncertainty. Because the status of the foetus is uncertain it can be argued that it should be treated as if it had the same rights as a baby. In an analogous way, if you were a hunter shooting at an object behind a bush which could be a man or a rabbit, you would be bound to treat it as if it was a man.

The argument from potential. This is well treated by Anne Fagot-Largeau (Fagot-Largeau 1996). In her view it is a weak argument because an entity with many different potentials is quite different from an entity which has actualised just one of many potentials (as an acorn is from a tree). Moreover, this argument can be used by anti-abortionists to argue for the rights of the foetus but also pro-abortionist to argue that a foetus may develop a disease and so should be aborted.

The argument from relationship. Many mothers will feel a foetus has moral rights in so far as they develop a relationship to it. For example, after quickening the mother forms more of a relationship and is often more reluctant to proceed to termination. Whereas contemporary Roman Catholic theologians dismiss ensoulment and the argument from potential, the argument from relationship is a key point for them. For they would argue that God forms a relationship at conception; as for example in Isaiah 44:2 "thus says God who made you, who formed you from the womb". While this is clearly an argument whose premise will not be shared by an atheist, its logic can, I hope, be understood.

The three possible positions for the doctor

I would like to look again at the three possible positions for the doctor and consider what effect they might have on the patient.

1. ***Rejection of dialogue.*** This is the option in which the doctor makes it known, say by a notice in the waiting room, that he will not see patients for termination. This position is strong on respect for the doctor's integrity. It gives a clear message to the patient. It gives the patient an example to model which is perhaps to stick up for her beliefs against the pressures of society, but it also models a refusal to engage in dialogue.

2. ***Private judgement.*** By this I mean a doctor who keeps his own moral judgement private and does not share it with the patient. As mentioned above, we all divide the rules we obey into those that apply to us and those we feel are universal. What happens to the doctor who perceives such a universal rule and fails to obey it? Firstly, he acts against the principle of respect for his own autonomy. Secondly, if we follow Aristotle, it will corrupt his moral character. Because, for Aristotle, the virtues are, as it were, the habits of doing good things, so that by doing good acts we become good. Conversely, by doing acts we believe are bad we will become bad. Thirdly, from a Kantian perspective, he would be dealing with the patient as a means and not an end. For to treat her as an end-in-herself is to share a rational moral argument with her and trust her judgement as a fellow rational human being. To refuse to share a rational argument with her is to fail to respect her capacity for reason and judgement, hence to treat her as a means (MacIntyre 1985). If the doctor refuses to share his ideas, he might be perceived by the patient as a doctor who thought himself so superior to, or so different from, her that he could not communicate with her.

3. *Moral dialogue.* So we come back to the third position: entering a dialogue with the patient.

A: Is moral dialogue possible in our society?

For a moral dialogue to be possible there are two requirements:

1. Shared words and concepts that form a more or less coherent framework and
2. Some means of using these words and concepts not only to describe moral choices but also to arrive at them.

Many would argue that moral dialogue is not possible in contemporary society because we do not share basic premises such as the existence of God or natural law. Nor do we share a common moral theory such as utilitarianism, or deontology or virtue theory, etc. As a result, our moral debates have a characteristically shrill tone as Alasdair MacIntyre points out (MacIntyre 1985). This shrill tone can characterise even our internal moral debates within our own selves. For example, a Roman Catholic GP faced with a woman facing abortion might hear two opposed internal voices, one saying "You should at all costs prevent this woman murdering her baby" while another says "You must respect her autonomy and her right to decide for herself".

I would like to look at two serious contemporary attempts to see if moral dialogue is possible. One is the Four Principles approach (Beauchamp & Childress 1983) and the other is the book of Alasdair MacIntyre "After Virtue" (MacIntyre 1985).

The Four Principles approach

These were first elaborated by Beauchamp and Childress at Geogetown University (Beauchamp & Childress 1983) and subsequently championed by Gillon (Gillon 1994). They consist of four unexceptional principles that most western doctors today would agree to:

1. The principle of respect for autonomy

2. Beneficence
3. Non-maleficence
4. Justice

They have been widely taught, especially in the USA, and so are familiar to many doctors. They certainly enable doctors to describe the grounds for their moral decisions in a way other doctors can understand.

There are however some limitations. The choice of principles appears arbitrary, and there is no reason to suppose that they include all the moral principles that a doctor might wish to consider. Beauchamp and Childress feel that the principles are strengthened because some of them can be derived from different moral theories (which is what they call coherentism). While this will help people familiar with different moral systems communicate, it does not to my mind increase their truth value. Finally, while the four principles may help people to communicate, because there is no way of weighing one up against another, they can only offer a framework for making or evaluating moral decisions (Finnis & Fisher 1994).

MacIntyre's "After Virtue"

MacIntyre certainly takes the problem of moral dialogue seriously (MacIntyre 1985) (chaps. 1&2). He claims that the moral concepts that we use today are like the ship-wrecked fragments of older and more consistent moral theories (in particular Aristotelian theories) and that, wrenched from their contexts, they are not only mutually incompatible but often left with little meaning.

To simplify, the history of ethics as he sees it goes a little like this. Aristotle (and his descendants, in particular the Thomists) had a metaphysical biology and ethics. All creatures strained towards an appointed end which was intrinsic in their nature. With the Enlightenment the metaphysical biology was abandoned. We no longer look for the end, purpose or, in Greek, 'telos' of biological phenomena but rather their cause. MacIntyre has no quarrel with that but holds that the enlightenment project of replacing an ethic linked to the proper end of man, a teleological ethic, with one based on reason alone, was misplaced. He holds that it was not only bound to fail but actually did fail. It can be seen to have actually failed because it has spawned a host of reason-based moral systems: utilitarianism, the philosophy of Kant, etc., which are not only incompatible but also successful and forceful critics of each other. It was bound to fail because ethics or virtues, as he sees them, are what lead man from the state he actually finds himself in to that state which is his proper end. Now for Aristotle that proper end was to be a free citizen of a Greek city state, and for Thomists it was to be a citizen of the heavenly city. While we clearly may not share those views of man's ideal state, we can agree with the argument that to think clearly about ethics we need to start by thinking about man's ends and purposes and not causes and reasons alone.

MacIntyre's positive suggestions are that virtues are the particular human qualities required to excel at and enjoy certain ways of life, such as being a doctor or a chess-player or a gardener. These must then be related to the narrative account of a whole life. Finally, the life itself must be lived within a social tradition.

How does this account help us understand the consultation with the patient? Firstly, the difficulty in talking about moral questions with people from a different background is well caught by his account. Secondly, we are very likely to recognise some of the concepts they do use, and, in so far as we share them from personal experience, or recognise them from our reading, we are better able to understand what our patient is saying. A patient, for example, might say "I could not get rid of my baby because he is alive". Even if she is a not a practising Catholic the origin of this concept can clearly be recognised. Thirdly, a woman whose concept of herself is within the narrative of a whole life, rather than broken fragments she feels beyond her control, will, at the least, approach the question of termination differently. Indeed, it could be argued that the role of motherhood only makes sense within the narrative concept of a whole life, and that a drastic shortage of "tales of motherhood" in modern culture has something to do with the large number of terminations. For how is a woman in a culture whose dominant stories are of woman as a "career girl" or as a "sex-object" to cope with being pregnant? Finally, his account has some resonance with Gilligan's classic feminist analysis (Gilligan 1993), based partly on interviews with women facing an abortion, that women's moral development (as op posed to men s) is characteristically based around relationships rather than rules.

As with the Four Principles, virtue theory gives us a way of thinking about moral actions but little content. It will not help us much in judging between right and wrong in a particular case. However, one area where it is helpful is in the distinction between the Nazi genocide and the current large number of terminations.

A digression: the distinction between the Nazi genocide and the current large number of terminations.

Aristotle thought that for an act to be virtuous it was necessary both for the action to be in itself virtuous and for it to be carried out for virtuous reasons. If a shopkeeper is kind to his customers in order to increase profit that is not virtue. The converse argument, to be found in Thomism, is that for an act to be sinful it is necessary both for it to be intrinsically wrong and for the person carrying out the act to know it is wrong. This explains why women who have terminations and gynaecologists who carry them out, are not corrupted by the acts they carry out, although, in my view, the acts are objectively wrong. For whereas the Nazi executioners were obviously and grossly corrupted by what they were doing, paradoxically that was because the moral upbringing they had received made them know that what they were doing was wrong, and it was this same knowledge that made them hide what they were doing. A modern gynaecologist doing terminations does not believe what he is doing is wrong, and for that reason his character is unaffected. Paradoxically again, it will be the Roman Catholic who feels he has been inveigled or pressured into terminations who will be corrupted, as I discussed in the section about private judgement above.

B: Ought we to engage in dialogue?

In Aristotle the word "ought" has only one meaning: to conform to the norms of the Greek city state (MacIntyre 1998). But in our own language "ought" has taken on two meanings;

a) A moral ought. Is it right or wrong, according to some moral perspective?
b) A socially normative ought. Is it the done thing in this society?

a) Looked at, for the moment, from the Roman Catholic perspective, there are some clear limitations to this dialogue. We have a clear duty to express the belief that the foetus does have rights and to express it not just in words but in action (Finnis & Fisher 1994). Not only should the abortion form not be signed, but the referral itself should not be made. This is because actions speak louder than words and, if the patient perceives you as referring her (even though you do not sign the abortion form), she may form the erroneous impression that you approve of termination. This stance involves inconvenience to our partners and means that, as soon as one judges that a woman definitely wants a termination, she must be asked to wait and see another partner for the actual referral.

b) Is it socially acceptable to engage in this sort of dialogue? Surprisingly it is commended by a leading pro-abortion group (Lloyd 1996) who states that those who are against abortion and engage in counselling should be open about their beliefs. In practice I have carried out such consultations for ten years without any complaint, and so it appears to be socially acceptable behaviour. However, some might still object that my counselling is not impartial. To this I would plead that impartiality is neither possible nor desirable. If I model openness, attentive listening and respect for the patient's autonomy and my own it may well influence them to follow these norms.

C: How should you engage in such a dialogue and is it effective?

This is something of an empirical as well as a moral question. From discussion with my colleagues it is clear that many GPs engage in this sort of dialogue. The only exception is the minority who believe that abortion is the mother's right on demand. For them there is no need to dialogue since they can just sign the abortion form. (Like all moral positions this one has its weak points; few such doctors would actually be happy with a termination on the ground of gender alone.)

Most doctors however do have a dialogue with the patient and naturally adapt the form of consultation they normally use when patients are facing a decision. For the RC doctor I have already pointed out two features designed to preserve his integrity:

1. Declare your own position;
2. Once it becomes clear that referral is decided upon, get another doctor to see the patient.

Clearly, while sharing one's own position may be desirable, it does not follow that it should be done at the outset, or insensitively. On the contrary, in my experience, with few exceptions, after the patient has talked for quite a long time, it feels quite appropriate to share one's own point of view with hers. Indeed, in the small market town where I practise people may already know my point of view and have chosen me for it. On the other hand, the position "if you need a referral you will need to see another GP" clearly has to be put early in the consultation to save the patient from the trauma of sharing her feelings twice.

In the early part of the consultation an opportunity must be given for the patient to share her thoughts and feelings. Paradoxically, in some cases, in order to do this, it may be necessary to tell the patient that a termination is easily available locally on the NHS, if she finally decides she wants one. Otherwise she may be so anxious about the possibility of a termination that her mind does not get beyond worry about this point.

Conventional advice might be to give the patient facts but not moral judgements. Unfortunately, facts are not so easily separated from judgements (MacIntyre 1985) (pages 83-84). In our context

89

the fact that the foetus has a heartbeat might be seen by the pro-choice lobby as moral blackmail, while the fact that abortion is readily available and post-abortion trauma rarely seen might equally be interpreted by pro-life groups as reflecting a moral stance. A more useful model is that in "Breaking bad news" by Robert Buckman (Buckman 1992) which deals with terminal care.

The analogy with terminal care.

In my experience, most of the time, what the patient is asking for is not a termination, but not to have been pregnant at all. This can account for the great urgency felt by some patients and their reluctance to think too clearly. In other words, the patient requesting a termination may be in a state of denial not unlike that of some terminal patients who do not believe they will die. In both cases breaking the denial can be traumatic. But in the case of termination the time frame is often only a couple of weeks and denial may well not be broken till after the termination. However, Buckman's model, somewhat simplified, is as follows:

1. find out what the patient knows,
2. find out what she wishes to know,
3. and close the gap.

Often the knowledge gap will include details of the local NHS availability for terminations. But it can be a comment like "I can't go through with a termination because I know my baby is alive", a comment that could be taken as a request for information about the biology and the ethical status of the foetus. Where possible an attempt should be made to get past the stage of denial since an ethical decision (on almost any basis) cannot be taken correctly if based on a false premise (I am not pregnant).

Summary

I have now had fifteen years' experience of consultations with women asking for terminations. In many cases the woman knows exactly what she wants, and no doctor is likely to alter her decision. Indeed, I suspect doctors grossly overestimate their capacity for altering patients' decisions. Nevertheless, that does not diminish their duty to use whatever influence they have responsibly. For the doctor who believes he has moral obligations to the foetus such consultations will continue to be a source of anguish. Nevertheless, on some occasions a moral dialogue is possible, perhaps because the mother shares a fragment of a moral system with her doctor. When dialogue can be undertaken I believe it is permissible to do so, though I have no quarrel with those who would not wish to do so. However, I believe it can model an attitude of unhurried listening, of respect for the patient's autonomy and of respect for the doctor's own integrity. In spite, or perhaps because, of the fact that I make my own views clear, I have found that many women who choose to opt for termination do continue their doctor-patient relationship with me. Only a handful, however, have changed their decisions after consulting me, and in all those cases strong ambivalence was present before the consultation.

References

Beauchamp, T. & Childress, J. 1983, Principles of biomedical ethics Oxford University Press, Oxford.
Buckman, R. 1992, How to break bad news Pan Books, London.
Donellan, C. 1997, The abortion debate Independence educational publishers, Cambridge.
Fagot-Largeau, A. 1996, "Abortion and arguments from potential," in The principles of health care ethics, R. Gillon, ed., John Wiley and sons, Chichester, pp. 577-586.
Finnis, J. & Fisher, A. 1994, "Theology and the four principles: a Roman Catholic view I," in The principles of health care ethics, R. Gillon, ed., John Wiley and sons, Chichester, pp. 31-45.
Gilligan, C. 1993, In a different voice Harvard University press, Cambridge Mass.
Gillon, R. 1986, Philosophical medical ethics John Wiley and sons, Chichester.
Gillon, R. 1994, ed., The principles of health care ethics John

Wiley and sons, Chichester.

Lloyd, L. 1996, "Abortion and health care ethics III." in The principles of health care ethics, R. Gillon, ed., John Wiley and sons, Chichester, pp.559-576.

MacIntyre, A. 1985, After Virtue, 2nd edn, Duckworth, London.

MacIntyre, A. 1998, A short history of ethics, 2nd edn, Routledge, London.

Mori, M. 1994, "Abortion and health care ethics I: a critical analysis of the main arguments," in Principles of health care ethics, R. Gillon, ed., Jon Wiley and sons, Chichester, pp. 53 1-546.

Shakespeare, T. 1998, "Choices and rights: eugenics, genetics and disability equality", Disability and Society, vol. 13, pp. 665-681.

The Independent. Obituary of Archbishop Johannes Dybla. 6-6. 26-7-2000. London. Ref Type: Newspaper

Wyatt, J. 1998, Matters of life and death IVP/CMF, London.

Essays

In a medical bookshop
Br J Gen Pract. 2007 Feb 1; 57(535): 161.

This summer I spent a day in central London walking around the area near my old medical school. My feet drifted to the old bookshop. There was still a floor of medical books, but no aisle was labelled "general practice". The assistant told me that there were a couple of racks at the back of the public health aisle.

When I tracked them down these racks were most disappointing. One was devoted to books teaching you how to pass exams or parts of exams. The other rack seemed equally dry – explanations of the health service, academic treatises and other worthy but unexciting books. These must be the books that are selling; books young doctors in training are actually buying. Perhaps they give us an insight into their priorities; to pass exams, to understand the subject.

But they were not the book for which I was looking. Indeed, until I failed to find it, I did not realise that I had been looking for it. A book with a title like "How to enjoy general practice and carry on enjoying it," that was the book for which I was looking.

Does such a book exist? If such a book were written it would have to talk about cricket. The fascination for the batsman is that every ball in every over is different. In the same way, the fascination of general practice for me is that, even after twenty years, each week at least, I see something new. I see something different; a new illness, a new way of responding to illness.

The glory of general practice is the people. The privilege is to see life from the perspective of such a wide variety of people; the ill and the well, the native and the immigrant. We are one of the few professions to be invited into the homes of almost all people. Often the pictures and decorations are filled with meaning which will be shared with us if we simply show a little interest. This business of seeing life from another person's point of view is called empathy; intellectual empathy if we understand their point of view, emotional empathy if we, so to speak, feel their feelings. This empathy needs to lead to action if it is not to be sterile. Fortunately, as GPs there is often something we can do, if only listening carefully and with respect. Empathy that leads to action, called in the Hebrew bible "chesed", this seems to me an essential virtue for general practice.

Most recently I have been privileged to work at the "Medical foundation for the care of victims of torture" writing medico-legal reports. Here I have met a man from Eritrea who was willing to risk torture in order meet with fellow Christians under the shade of a tree at noon. I have met a shepherd from the desert who had never been in a town before, yet had to give his story a shape that would be understandable to a home office official. I have met, alas, with the Home Office and its "culture of disbelief" and its policy of driving "failed asylum seekers" into destitution. I have also come across the stories of many individuals and groups who have helped.

This experience, painful as it is at times, has re-enforced my sense of privilege at sharing in the stories of so many people. So, in my experience, general practice can remain enjoyable – so long as the empathic feelings and understandings generated by our work are followed by action and not squandered in inactivity or cynicism.

A modest proposal 2008 (unpublished)
(After Jonathan Swift)

From a speech by the Home Secretary 2020

Identity cards have been a great success in re-enforcing our British sense of identity and enabling us to police our borders more effectively. However, their value has been damaged by the criminal actions of some members of our society – and let me reassure people that the government will pursue such criminals with all possible vigour. It is therefore time to consolidate the benefits that a secure identity has brought to our society.

First, I must mention – if only in passing – the pusillanimous proposals of the opposition. Their suggestion was that babies should have a microchip inserted under the skin at birth, much as happens to puppies. This was simply too open to fraud and it failed to take advantage of the latest modern technology in miniature telephones. Moreover, they did not win over the medical profession, so that their proposal involved all babies being micro chipped at the vets; an idea understandably unpopular with some members of the public.

This is why our Government is keen to involve general practitioners in the earliest stages of these exciting new proposals. For what we suggest is nothing less than this; inserting a telephone chip into the brain of all babies at birth. Now here is a proposal which will need the technical skills of our wonderful British doctors. The procedure is simple and quite safe. It has already been widely implemented in the Ukrainian Republic – surely what the Ukrainians can do we can do better. The chip will be inserted immediately after birth through the baby's anterior fontanelle straight into the ventricles of the brain. Once there it will remain for life and very soon it becomes almost impossible to remove. Not only will it be useful as an identity tag, it will have many other purposes.

For example, we plan to use it to store the individual's health record. Every time they go to see their GP or other doctor the patients will wear headphones which will update the microchip, "as the GP types into his computer." Naturally the information that can be stored will not be limited to health. The head of Her Majesty's Revenue and Customs is very excited at the possibility of storing all his tax data within the taxpayer's own head. The banks could do without smart cards or PIN numbers – simply insert your head into the cash machine. The cash machine could dispense summary justice to fraudsters – though perhaps this is a step which should be further examined before we legislate.

The real excitement of our proposals is that the government could simply telephone the citizens at its leisure and in the privacy of the individual's own head. We could consult citizens widely and easily on a variety of proposals. A telephone call from the government could remind citizens to fill in a tax form, to vote, or perform some other civic duty. All citizens could be told to stay indoors at certain specific times so that the police could literally clean the streets of undesirable people who either lacked the microchips or had chosen to forfeit their citizenship by ignoring the Government's instruction.

The true vision is that our nation could become more that an accumulation of individuals, but instead a true super-organism; a single united "Cyberpeople." Under the leadership of our heroic Prime Minister we could then overtake other nations not only on the economic but also the military fronts. Britain could once again be great. There would be no need to waste resources on parliaments or democracy when our Leader could directly communicate with every citizen. Instead we could devote all our resources to rebuilding our greatness so that one day – a not too distant day perhaps – we could regain the liberty that we had so willingly abandoned for a short time.

"The Human Condition" Unpublished

The Belgian surrealist Magritte made a well-known painting which he cryptically called "The Human Condition" (1933.) It is one of a series on this subject to which he returned throughout his life. It depicts a landscape, perhaps a suburban park, framed by a window. Part of the landscape is obscured by a canvas on an easel which depicts the very landscape it is also hiding. While the purpose of the painting is to startle the viewer and make him think, so that it can legitimately bear many interpretations, I wish to expand on only one interpretation in this essay. The painted canvas within the painting both obscures part of the view, a tree, and depicts it. Is the artist saying that this is the essential nature of the concepts with which we understand the world? They, on the one hand, help us to understand the world and, on the other obscure or limit our understanding of the reality which they are trying to depict. For example, while the concept of depression does helpfully enable to understand and help another person, it can often prevent us from perceiving the unique complexity of their experience. It is a matter of wonder that the human brain – about the size and texture of a generous plate of porridge – can usefully understand the outside world at all. Magritte, surrealist and Marxist as he was, is rather pointing us to an essential limitation of our understanding. The message of this interpretation of the painting, then, is essentially negative. Every time we understand something we inevitably use words which by their previous usage, the baggage they carry, limit and restrict the very thing we are trying to understand. As Elliot put it in the first quartet "Burnt Norton" (written in 1935);

.... Words strain,
    Crack and sometimes break, under the burden,
Under the tension, slip, slide, perish,
Decay with imprecision, will not stay in place,
Will not stay still.

In the consultation we have an advantage over the landscape painter. The person we are trying to understand, unlike a hill or a tree, can talk back to us. Inevitably, like the landscape painter, we start by using our concepts, our pre-judged ideas, our prejudices, if you like. It is by applying these pre-judged ideas that we build up a picture of the person before us. By applying these ideas layer upon layer as a painter might apply his oil paints, we reach a picture of the person before us that, we hope, shows some likeness. At the same time, as Magritte is pointing out, that picture, flawed or not, is never the original likeness, but a representation of it and this limitation must always be borne in mind. However, in the consultation the subject can himself guide us along. In the consultation we feed-back to the patient the concepts we have used and he corrects and refines them further until he agrees that they are a good enough depiction of what he is trying to convey. Indeed, in some consultations this is a principal element, as many people will say that "they do not know what they want to say until they have said it to somebody." That is to say in many consultations our main aim is helping people to tell their own stories, to make sense of their own lives. One clue that this may have been the case is when people say as they are leaving, just when we feel we have been no use to them, "thank you for listening." The human condition, then, is perhaps not as bleak as an initial response to Magritte's painting would have us believe.

As water is to fish, so is society to people.
Br J Gen Pract. 2011 Jan 1; 61(582): 74–75.
doi: 10.3399/bjgp11X549144

Looking down from a bridge onto a lake with Koi carp, I can see them moving sinuously through the water. Their progress appears natural, effortless. If I could ask the carp, would they be aware that they are swimming in water? I think not. Maybe they would talk about their own ability at swimming, their long hours of practice, that clever signature flick of their tail and never mention the element in which they live. Perhaps fish only become aware of the existence of water when they are taken out of it; are landed gasping on the river bank by a fisherman. Then they realise its importance and know that, if they are not returned within minutes, they will die. So it is for us. People, especially modern people, see themselves as independent actors who forge their own lives, who create their own meaning out of their lives. Yet take a man out of society into solitary confinement and in short order a number will go quite mad. Those who remain sane, and some have survived solitary confinement for years, sometimes do so supported by a sense of the justness of their cause, of a society out there supporting them. Others engage in elaborate rituals of exercise, memory and prayer to impose order.
We know why water is so important for fish, but why is society so important for people? Clearly, we are to a greater extent social beings than modern models might have us think. One reason is that many of things we take for granted are actually social goods. By social goods I mean things that only exist because they, or belief in them, are shared by a whole society. Language, for example is a social good. It only exists, is only useful for communication,

because a whole society shares the language. It already exists before we are born; the individual does not create it. We cannot ascribe arbitrary meanings to words. Money is also a social good. Money only has value because individuals in a society share a belief in its value. If they lose this belief (as in societies with hyper-inflation), the value disappears. Witchcraft in some societies works in exactly the same way, as I learnt when I worked in Central Africa. If all individuals in the society believe in it, then the effects of witchcraft are real. An outsider saying that witchcraft does not exist is as completely ignored as a stranger to England who said that paper money was worthless. Finally, power in most of its forms is again a social good. It depends for its existence on the belief of both the rulers and the ruled. When this belief wanes, revolution becomes possible and those who were powerful can become powerless.

(Conversely the power of general practitioners is largely informal. It is only as we use it on behalf of our patients by writing to housing authorities, benefits agencies, hospitals and so on that it becomes real. If we do not use it withers away.)

If we take seriously this understanding of people as not only incarnate in a body and possessing a mind, but also enmeshed in society, does this have any implications for general practice? If we were to treat this question systematically we would need to consider its implications for the patient, the doctor and his engagement with society and politics. In this essay, however, I only want to mention some random examples. Teaching GP trainees, they often need coaching to elicit the social world of their patients; relationships, occupations, position in society. All general practitioners need to decide to what extent they will get involved in claims for benefits. This is a particularly topical question right now when the government is aiming to get most people under fifty off long term incapacity benefit.

These people are hitting our consulting rooms on a daily basis because these changes have profound implications for them. The need for a new social network is perhaps most acutely felt by refugees and asylum seekers; I have reviewed their needs for primary care elsewhere (Vernon and Feldman 2006). Other people who need to find a new social group would be recently released prisoners, drug addicts who wish to give a drug up they are used to with its attendant live style and, more prosaically, the depressed, especially those with post-natal depression.

The social nature of people is used therapeutically by a strand of narrative medicine described by John Launer (Launer 2002). Into the consultation between the doctor and the patient, the doctor introduces other people from the patient's social world. For example, where the patient has a long-term partner, it is possible to ask, "What do you think your partner would say?" This can break the log-jam in a consultation and at its least can be illuminating. We can find out that the partner thinks that the patient is making a fuss, in which case they may be right; that the partner has not been told, which highlights communication issues, or that the partner has specific health beliefs or anxieties which can then be addressed. For many people in our country today that social world includes a creator God, and therefore religious and spiritual concerns can be raised in this way.

I would like to give an example of such a consultation which occurred between a junior anaesthetist and a patient many years ago. I think it shows the potential of this consultation technique. The anaesthetic SHO was asked to see an old man on the ward with intolerable pain due to metastatic prostate cancer in the spine. He inserted an epidural and started a local anaesthetic infusion, thus relieving the immediate pain, then began to talk to the old man. It was night and the ward was quiet.

It became clear that the old man was heartbroken because he was estranged from his alcoholic daughter. He longed to be reconciled with her before he died, but could see no reasonable prospect for this. He also felt guilty because he had neglected his God. He felt it was no good turning to God at the end after a lifetime of ignoring him. When asked if he would forgive his daughter if she returned he said that of course he would; the longing could be seen on his face. I asked him if he thought God too would forgive him if he turned to him. He burst into tears as this point came home to him. As it happens his back pain did not recur although the epidural infusion was taken down. He was reconciled to his daughter who was seen pushing him round the hospital in a wheelchair. Why did the pain not recur? I do not know. Pain is not just a pure sensation, but one that comes, as it were with a meaning attributed from the beginning. Physical interruption of the sensation by an anaesthetic drug can ease the pain, but so can re-attribution of a different meaning. This pain in his mind had something to do with his rift with his daughter. Maybe, with the rift healed, the pain was less of an overwhelming threat. (Examples in daily practice are less dramatic, but we have all seen patients after a heart attack who interpret every ache in their chest which they would previously have ignored, as angina. They will respond to careful listening and re-assurance that these sensations have no sinister meaning, but are normal.)

Our view of society will also have an effect on the sort of doctor we strive to be; one the one hand, a doctor who gets involved in the local community, a Doctor Finlay, or at the other extreme a bureaucratic, Stakhanovite ticker of QOF boxes. Finally, how we view society will have an effect on how keen we are to engage with politics at all levels. If man's very self is embedded in society, is the striving for social justice integral to the role of the doctor?

References

Launer, J. 2002. *Narrative-based Primary Care* Oxford, Radcliffe Medical Press.
Vernon, G. & Feldman, R. Refugees in Primary Care: from looking after to working together.
http://www.networks.nhs.uk/uploads/09/08/refugeesupdate4with_t ables.doc accessed 15/08/09 .

Between 'thisness' and quiddity: The place of the GP.
Br J Gen Pract 2013: DOI: 10.3399/bjgp13X669284

The role of the general practitioner is to apply his knowledge of medicine, science, the arts, to an individual patient in front of him. Two philosophical concepts from the 13th century can help us here. "Thisness," "haecceity" is the characteristics of the being that make it that particular being. The thisness of my dog lies in the way she wags her tail, prefers ball games even to food, twitches her nose; all the things which make her just herself and not another dog. All things have thisness, not just people and dogs. A rock will have an individual essence which makes it just this rock and not another one. The 13th century philosopher Duns Scotus popularised the notion of haecceity, adapting it from Aristotle, and he has had many admirers down the centuries, including the German philosopher Martin Heidegger (who in 1915 wrote his habilitation thesis on the philosophy of Duns Scotus.) But it was the Victorian poet and Jesuit, Gerald Manley Hopkins, who coined "thisness" as an English word meaning haecceity. He memorably uses the concept in his poem "As kingfishers catch fire;"(1;2)

Each mortal thing does one thing and the same:

....

..................., *myself* it speaks and spells,
Crying *What I do is me: for that I came*

Quiddity is in some ways the opposite. This is those characteristics a dog shares with other dogs which make it a dog, a table with other tables that make it a table. Now science studies precisely this, the things we share in common so that a treatment that works for one man may work for all. As general practitioners we take a treatment that works in general and see if it is appropriate in a particular person. Evidence based medicine acknowledges this when it says that you should consider whether the patient in front of you is like the patients in the trial; in terms of age, sex, and place of care (that is hospital or primary care.) These categories do belong to the thisness of the patient before you, as opposed to the quiddity, but they are poor categories. By poor categories I mean they do not take you very far in describing the particular person in front of you and therefore in deciding whether that particular treatment will suit him. We need a richer picture of the individual human being. I have written earlier of the numerous and conflicting meta-narratives with which post-modern man may seek simultaneously to understand the world(3). It is certainly worth becoming aware of these by listening carefully to the patient – by eliciting their thoughts, beliefs and expectations as we tell our trainees. However, the privileged way to access the thisness of a patient is by dialogue; together we can struggle to work out if the proposed treatment is a suitable treatment for this patient. Our thisness does not lie in the mind alone but in our social role and in our body. Can this person open this pill-bottle; can he read or remember instructions, what are his pharmaco-genetics? This dialogue is clearly an iterative process; when we talk to the patient we move between quiddity and thisness, the general and the particular, until we agree on a best course of action.

Interestingly, in designing treatments, modern western medicine starts from quiddity whereas traditional therapeutic systems start from thisness; they consider what is individual about the patient and base their treatment choice on this. For example, according to Michel Foucault, the medieval Western physician would design his treatment starting from the health beliefs of his client(4).

The motto of the Royal College of General Practitioners is "Cum Scientia, Caritas." "Scientia," in this context means knowledge, knowledge about the general properties of things, their quiddity. Caritas simply means love. Love implies not only grasping the thisness of the person in front of us, but choosing to act in a way that respects this. To grasp the thisness of the person in front of us we need both intellectual and emotional empathy. Intellectual empathy means understanding their situation from their point of view. Emotional empathy means feeling the emotions they feel. In the jargon of psycho-analysis this is called counter-transference. In every day practice it simply means that I become aware that I am feeling anxious or angry or depressed and realising that this is a clue to what the patient is feeling. Love is not love that is empathy alone, it must lead to action, but action now attuned to the world of our patient rather than our own.

To summarise the role of the general practitioner is to apply his knowledge, which relates to humankind in general, its quiddity, to the individual before him in all his glorious thisness and eccentricity. This is a very general description of which I have only sketched some consequences here. However, it means that we have a job that is unique and irreplaceable. The more our scientific knowledge increases the more this role will be needed. At a time when some GPs feel disorientated, this role is something clearly needed which we are good at and can be proud of. Of course, general practitioners do many other things; running practices, rationing the health service and so on. But we should not be seduced into making these more important than what I see as our prime and irreplaceable role; interpreting quiddity to thisness.

Reference List

(1)   Hopkins G. Poems and Prose of Gerald Manley Hopkins. London: Penguin Books; 1953.

(2)   Bates T. Duns Scoutus and the problem of universals. London: Continuum; 2010.

(3)   Vernon G. Essay - What is man? BJGP 2003;53:504-5.

(4)   Foucault M. Naissance de la Clinique. Paris: Presses Universitaire de France; 1963.

Darwin's dream (unpublished)

(In the following short story Charles Darwin is the famous scientist, author of "On the Origin of Species by Means of Natural Selection". Professor Florence Cady of the Avian Behavioural Unit at the University of Belfast is a fictional character)

After a copious Victorian lunch, Charles Darwin retired to his study at Down House. He had allowed himself a glass of sherry. Although he had told his wife, Emma that he must return straightaway to his work on beetles, he sat down. His eyes felt heavy. The eyelids drooped. Soon he was asleep.

In his dream he saw a woman climb into his study through a window which had been left ajar, for it was a warm spring day. Because he was dreaming, he felt no surprise at this unusual mode of entry. The woman was dressed mannishly, in country clothes, yet there was an intensity in her eyes, a purpose in her step, that marked her out as a retired professor. She cleared her throat and bowed formally.

"Let me introduce myself, I am professor Florence Cady."

 Darwin motioned her to sit down. On the professor's shoulder was a pigeon. As the professor sat down, the pigeon hopped on to the table besides Darwin and started to preen herself. On the little table was a miniature portrait of Annie, the eight year old daughter whom Darwin and Emma had lost the year before. Since that loss a silence had fallen upon the household. He and Emma rarely spoke. They blamed themselves; they blamed each other for the death of their daughter. Darwin himself was often ill; his mother had died when he was eight. Had she inherited this illness from him? Darwin and Emma were cousins; was inbreeding the problem? Inbreeding was a subject he would later investigate.

Because of this silence Darwin welcomed the professor's company. Besides he was often troubled by dreams in which eminent Victorians berated him about his great book, "The Origin of Species", pointing out its dangers the nation's faith and morals, so much so that Darwin was to delay another decade before he published his book. But the professor looked more fun than the average visitor; the pigeon marked her out as a practical naturalist rather that a theologian. Besides Darwin had not met many female academics. Professor Cady opened her mouth, "No, Charles, your theories don't solve the riddle."

"Dear professor," Darwin responded, "by all means let us discuss my theory. Where does it fail?"

"If I may quote from the book which you are writing, and which, coming (as I do in your dream) from Belfast in the twentieth century, I have had the privilege to study;

"As many more individuals of each species are born than can possibly survive; and as, consequently, there is a frequently recurring struggle for existence, it follows that any being, if it vary however slightly in any manner profitable to itself, under the complex and sometimes varying conditions of life, will have a better chance of surviving, and thus be *naturally selected*. From the strong principle of inheritance, any selected variety will tend to propagate its new and modified form.""

"You have put it better than I have yet been able to do," interjected Darwin.

"Please look at my pigeon. When has she pushed anyone aside in the struggle for existence? On the contrary she risks her life incubating her eggs and even protecting them against predators."

"The food she eats is food another creature could have eaten," countered Darwin. He settled himself into his armchair; he was beginning to enjoy this debate. Turning to his left he saw the pigeon preening herself and his daughter Annie looking up from the photograph with that look of wonder that children have; as if they are seeing something for the first time. Caught unawares a tear rolled down his cheek. He left it untouched, hoping his strange visitor would not notice it.

"Dear Charles," said the professor, "the loss of your daughter has burnt your heart and your mind, so that now the world appears black. From that blackness, you see only the survival of the fittest. Yet you could add another sentence to your book; "Among social insects, the tendency to co-operate will improve the chances of survival for the colony. Thus, co-operation too will be naturally selected and inherited."

Darwin thought. "Selection may be applied to the family, as well as the individual, and thus may gain the desired end." He paused, "Yes, I get your point. Of course, the cells in an organ like my liver co-operate, they are right now breaking down the alcohol from the sherry which I have just drunk, but all the cells in it have the same genes. The ants in a colony have different genes, yet they too cooperate; selection can occur not only at the level of the individual, but also the group. One colony of ants may be more successful than another; that colony survives even though some of the individuals are sterile."

"You have got my point," the professor agreed. "And not only the social insects; the care a mother pigeon shows for her chicks, the time at which she chooses to stop feeding them when fledged so that they are forced to start flying, all these traits of love are inherited too. That tear rolling down your cheek is inherited from your father, Robert; remember how he cried when your mother died."

The professor rose to leave. "I have learnt more from you in this dream than from many visits to learned societies," Darwin said politely as he saw her back to the window. When the professor had climbed out of the window, she was surrounded by a flock of pigeons that had been waiting for her on the lawn. Darwin's tears overflowed to see the affection which the birds seemed to feel for her. When his eyes had cleared the professor and her pigeons had disappeared. He sat down again. "Perhaps both the instinct for survival and for care is inherited; I shall have to rewrite my book yet again." But when he woke memory of what the professor had said fled rapidly from him. He only managed to scribble down one sentence before it had all gone; "selection may be applied to the family, as well as the individual, and thus may gain the desired end."

(That sentence did appear in "The Origin of Species" when it was published in 1859, but few people noticed it. "Group selection" as a theory to explain the evolution of eusocial insects was not published till 2010, one hundred and fifty years after the original publication.)

Sources

Martin A. Nowak, Corina E. Tarnita, Edward O. Wilson, "The evolution of eusociality" Nature 466: 1057-1062 (2010)

Edward O. Wilson, "The social conquest of the earth" Livewright, New York 2012

A light bulb moment
BJGP 2016 Jul;66(648):379

Many years ago, when I was a GP trainer, I went to on a visit to an old lady. She was recently bereaved, arthritic, not far from the end of life herself. In those days we did more chronic visits, so that the content of the visit was as much personal as medical. With me I had my current registrar. She was bright, enthusiastic, knowledgeable. As we left the old lady asked me the change a light bulb in the kitchen; her hands were not up to it. I changed the light bulb; it was the work of moments.

As we got back into the car I saw a look of thunder on my registrar's face. She had not trained for seven years in order to change light bulbs, she told me. If she'd wanted to change light bulbs she could have trained as an electrician, or even – yes, she would come out with it, as a nurse or an occupational therapist. I kept my peace; turned to other matters. Middle-aged now, probably a mother, still, I hope, a GP, these days she probably changes light bulbs for patients without even noticing that she's doing it.

But what I could have said then, what I bit back because it would not have helped at that moment, was the following;

"You trained for seven years to acquire more; to acquire more skills, to acquire the status and respect due to a doctor. You did not train for seven years to become less; you did not train for seven years to become less human."

Towards a virtue ethics for general practice (Three short stories)
I would claim little managerial or administrative skill. But I joined a well-run practice. I could no more read a balance sheet when I joined than when I left. Yet I was a partner for many years and, as senior partner for the last few, I simply continued established practices. The practice aimed to look after the patients first and only secondly employed staff to ensure that the health service paid

us for everything we had done. Strange as it may seem, this worked; the patients were looked after and the practice thrived. This is, perhaps, a good place to record my gratitude to my preceding senior partners; Drs John Tasker, James Rawes, Simon Jackson and Malcolm Slack and also to Mrs. Anne Taylor our long-standing practice manager. One innovation which I introduced shortly after arrival was the practice annual report. The head of each department; dispensary, reception, the nurses, the doctors and so on, wrote an annual report on the work of her department and the whole was edited into one report. Mortality and morbidity statistics, for example the average BP of our hypertensives, the average Hba1c of our diabetics, was added. Many of the staff read it with interest; they learnt to respect each other's work. The lift to morale was worth the small effort involved. When we started, I believe we were the first in Essex. We stopped writing an annual report when QOF was introduced in 2012 as, effectively, a national system of reporting was then introduced.

(QOF (Quality and Outcomes Framework) is a performance management system introduced in 2012. Its purpose was to improve the care of a number of diseases by the systematic collection of evidence leading to payment by targets. Overnight GPs started to spend minutes of every consultation on ticking boxes. The expectation, which I shared, was that on obvious drop in IHD (Ischaemic Heart Disease) mortality would follow. This has not proved to be the case. IHD mortality has continued to fall in the UK at the same rate as before. The reason for this is unclear. One factor was however predicted at the outset. A GP columnist in "Pulse" (a popular GP magazine) who uses the pen-name "Tony Copperfield" wrote of QOF in the week of its inception, "it is a cheat's charter".

The pressure to meet targets revolutionised within a year the way blood pressure was recorded in General Practice. Where office BPs (BPs measured in the General Practice) had been used, we moved to home BPs measured by the patients because these are lower and more likely to meet the targets. It is also true that that they correlate better with IHD outcomes and are therefore, probably, a more appropriate measurement. One lesson of QOF for me is that the person measuring a variable must not be the person who is rewarded for reaching a target based on that variable; there must be two separate people, separately paid. However, distortion of the evidence cannot be the sole factor, for QOF lead to a huge increase in the use of statins, increases that had been predicted to lead to measurable increases in the fall in IHD, but which, similarly failed to do so.)

Below are three short stories set in general practice. Each illustrates a virtue needed to work as a GP; compassion in "The Lost sheep", practical common sense in "Innocent as doves", perseverance in "The Lazy doctor"; in "The right view of time" the title speaks for the contents[5]. Virtue ethics, originating with Aristotle and developed in our day by Alistair McIntyre, I have discussed at length above in the article "Can there be a moral dialogue between Doctor and Patient?" For virtue ethics to have a content; to usefully describe a way of life, we need to know the virtues particular to that way of life. These stories, then, are about some of the virtues required for general practice.

The lost sheep
BJGP Br J Gen Pract 2017; 67 (664): 517

Sarah was, in many ways, the archetypal lost sheep. Brought up by poor immigrant parents, battered by her father as a girl, she never seemed to have a chance. For years we hardly saw her, hidden, as it were, in a back room by her widowed mother. She was on drugs; heroin, cannabis, anything she could lay her hands on. Then in her thirties she vanished for a long stretch inside one of Her Majesty's Prisons. She returned more sinister than before, dragging an air of menace through our streets. She befriended and ruthlessly exploited the other drifters and drunks of our small town.

She took to haunting the surgery, demanding drugs. She would bring her sad, battered, tattooed face up close and request diazepam, co-proxamol, tramadol. She demanded treatment for the intolerable pain in her heart. She searched in vain for a cardiologist, a respiratory specialist, for anybody who would agree to further tests. Each consultation was a game of chess; would some new referral, some harmless tablet, get her out of the consulting room before she turned violent? I often thought that that

---

[5] The most striking story about this, far better than mine, "The right view of time" is in Matthew 18:22 where Jesus, on his way to heal the daughter of Jairus, who had died – a crash call if ever there was one – stops to heal a woman who had been suffering from menorrhagia for twelve years.

might be how I would die; that she would get out her knife and kill me. Yet she was the one who died.

We never barred her from the list. She did not misbehave in the waiting room; her worst crime was once taking away a bunch of flowers. Her presence gave a message to the other patients there. All were welcome. Whatever your troubles, you could come to this surgery.

The last time I saw her, she wished me well for my retirement. A week or two later she was dead. She had died in the local hospital. The day after her death came a fax setting forth all the circumstances of that death. No hospital had done that in thirty years. Something had gone wrong in the hospital; the rank smell of a cover-up hung in the air. I spoke to the police, but they were not interested.

We mourned for her, for the lost sheep has a value for the rest of the flock. She enables the shepherd to act out, to demonstrate, his sacrificial care for all. But she also sets limits to that care. For those who do not wish to share the waiting room with the world's down and outs can get up and go. They are free to leave and seek care elsewhere. The shepherd does not exclude them; they exclude themselves.

Be cunning as snakes and yet innocent as doves (unpublished)

Doctor Jones was a GP in a leafy suburb of Bristol. Drug addicts rarely came his way; most of the practice list were commuters. Yet one grey autumn day a thickset middle-aged man did arrive at the practice reception desk. He limped in, his face a grimace of pain. He gave his name, using a soft American accent, as Jack Smith. The receptionists were kind people, cat lovers, collectors of waifs and strays. They greeted the man politely, provided him with a pair of metal crutches for his painful leg, squeezed him into an extra appointment slot with Dr Jones.

Some half an hour later Mr. Smith limped into Dr Jones consulting room making a great show of his pain. He was just in the area for a day, he said; he had forgotten to bring his pain-killers. Something about the man alerted Dr Jones; the demand for pain killers was too transparent. When Dr Jones enquired further it became all too clear that the man wanted only opioid type pain killers; Distalgesic, codeine or pethidine. Offers of other pain killers, paracetamol based or anti-inflamatories were rejected out of hand. Once the situation was clear to him, Dr Jones told the man that he would not be prescribing any opioids. Mr. Smith suddenly became angry. He said, brandishing his crutch in his right hand; "I'll make you feel the pain I'm feeling."

Dr Jones had to think quickly. He had no wish to be hit by a long piece of metal. By his left hand was a red panic button. If he hit this a loud noise would emerge, but it might be a while before any help came, for, until that day, the alarm button had only ever been pressed in error in that surgery. Moreover, the loud noise might well startle the drug addict, who would have plenty of time to hit him before help came. Dr. Jones spoke to the man, as if to suggest a compromise; "I can see this is a difficult problem. Can I phone a colleague to ask for his help?" He did not wait for agreement, but rang Dr. Doos on the internal phone. Now Dr Doss was, in fact, a young doctor being trained by Dr. Jones. Moreover, he was quick on the uptake, streetwise as you might say, six foot four and a onetime Olympic rower. When he heard Doctor Jones asking him for advice about a patient, he understood immediately that something was going wrong in Doctor Jones consulting room. He abandoned what he was doing and came straight into Dr Jones's room. As soon as his massive six foot four frame filled the door it was clear to the three men that the game was over. Mr. Smith simply stood up. Without further ado he walked out of the consulting room without using the crutches and without a limp. Dr Jones thanked his registrar and asked the practice manager to warn the other practice in town. They continued their afternoon surgery.

The Lazy doctor (unpublished)

Mike Roberts was a lazy doctor. He worked on the wards of City Central Hospital. It was not that he was born lazy; if that had been the case, he would never have qualified as a doctor. No, the inspiration had come to him after qualification. It came from within; it was not inspired by any particular example. He simply realised that most jobs could be left undone. Left undone, somebody else would do them for him. The doctors were in the middle of a strike. Mike had no strong feelings on the matter, but he took it as an opportunity to do even less work than usual.

His job this morning was to summarise a huge pile of notes belonging to patients who had recently been discharged; patients he had never personally seen. The pile had grown to gigantic proportions over the last two weeks of the strike. A quick inspection of the office enabled him to identify an empty drawer at the bottom of a filing cabinet. That would make a suitable resting place for the notes while he had a nice cup of coffee. Nobody could expect him to summarise them all; if anybody complained, the strike could be blamed. He had just put on the kettle when the ward clerk came in. "It's that GP again, he rings every day for Peter Smith's summary, he wants to speak to you."

Mike could see Peter Smith's notes on top of the pile. He would do anything rather than speak to that insufferable GP again. "Tell him I'm doing them now," he told the ward clerk. It would be less trouble summarising the one set of notes, than getting hassled by that old fashioned GP yet again. While he drank his coffee, a latte macchiato, he summarised the one set of notes and shoved the others to the back of the filing cabinet. Then he sat back in his chair; he was ready for the ward round, fresh as a morning daisy.

Mike Roberts, the lazy doctor, who does not care a hoot about patients, gave in to the old fashioned GP's persevering requests; perseverance works.

The right view of time (unpublished)

I was working then as a junior anaesthetist. Anaesthetists rarely admire surgeons unreservedly, for we work with them on a daily basis and see their strengths and weaknesses from close by. As the proverb has it, "No man is a hero to his valet." But for Davina Ball, I did have great admiration for, to my mind, she had the right view of time.

Surgeons are not known for their human qualities so that Davina stood out all the more because she treated her patients as people. Don't get me wrong – we need surgeons – strong, decisive, and unafraid to cut the human body, as this story will show. But Davina stood out as human and this did not make her popular with her peers. They vaguely disliked and resented her because she had something they lacked; her promotions came slower than theirs. If a patient she had seen years ago stopped her in the corridor, she would talk to them. People came to her with their troubles; she could listen for half an hour and not look at her watch. As a result she was often late. We anaesthetists and theatre staff liked her so much that we worked round her. I remember asking her husband how he coped with her constant lateness. "She was like that when I married her," he replied, "I knew what I was taking on."

But when I say that she had the right view of time, I mean that she was open to the moment; sometimes it meant that she was late, but she could also work efficiently, even ruthlessly. One day we were called to a ward where a woman was vomiting bright red blood; it was pumping out of her mouth. Maybe they called us straight from theatre because, as I remember it, we were the first to arrive. Her pulse was already weak. Davina took charge and the two of us pushed the bed through the corridors of the hospital. We took the bed right into the operating theatre bypassing the anaesthetic room. I gave her a tiny amount of thiopentone so that she lost consciousness and I intubated her. We transferred the patient onto the operating table. Davina operated with great rapidity, finding and sewing up the bleeding vessel in her stomach within minutes. The patient survived, but only because of Davina's decisive action and disregard of protocol; one could not imagine many of her colleagues dispensing with porters and pushing the bed themselves.

For Aristotle a virtue is a mean between two extremes. A right view of time, then, is neither rigid punctuality nor an endless going with the flow but the right mean between the two.

Teaching "Evidence based medicine"

Before the MSc course, I had come across David Sackett's book "Evidence based Medicine". After many years in general practice it came to me as an intoxicating shaft of light. I went on a week's course run by Professor Greenhalgh, and then I taught EBM myself on an occasional basis. The following two pieces were published during that period. The first is a version of a portfolio item on the MSc written with Dr Graham Wheatley, a colleague on the course.

In the article, statins are used as an example. They were coming in at that time. In the practice our partner Dr Gillian Graves drew our attention to the 4S paper on the benefits of statins in secondary prevention and we became early adopters of this treatment. At one point we even gained a boost to our prescribing budget from the health authority for this purpose.

How to learn and teach statistics for EBM
Education for Primary Care 2001, written with Graham Wheatley

Context
Medical teachers face the problem that doctors have difficulty learning mathematical concepts the usual way. This is becoming a more common problem with the increasing use of EBM. While not in reality innumerate (they all passed "O" level or GCSE maths and can do household accounts), they behave as if they were. Partly this is due to disuse atrophy since it can be twenty years since they have dealt with an equation. For some there is a clear and obvious phobia about numbers which must date back to negative experiences at school. The trick is clearly to take the reluctant doctor, by a circuitous route avoiding numbers, until the doctor is over the hurdle without noticing he has jumped it. In more technical terms we face the problem of androgogy in the specific instance of numerical concepts.

A striking example of teaching statistics in a different way took place at the fourth London workshop on EBM. Participants were experiencing difficulty attempting to learn statistics about therapeutic trials. Dr. Celia Duff (of the Anglia and Oxford office of the NHS executive) then divided people into two small sub-groups of four people each. Each group had to come up with tabloid headlines for or against a trial of nicotine patches based on the figures she had given us. When shouting slogans at each other had brought us no nearer agreement, we were ready to follow her through the definitions of statistics used in therapeutic trials (such as number needed to treat). Interest had been generated from a need for a language in which to talk about therapeutic trials; statistics then supplied it. Computation was introduced gradually, avoiding memories of school failures.

Aim

The aim, then, is to develop a new way of teaching numerical concepts to doctors that by-passes the fear of mathematics and the partial innumeracy which so many experience. We are looking for a way not only to teach them statistics, but to teach them how to teach it.

Learning Method

We have developed a method which we call the four step method.

Table 1

The four step model.

	Steps	Origins
Step 1	Create the learning need	Wlodkowski[1] and Knowles[2]
Step 2	Transmitting knowledge	
Step 3	Check that the teacher has taught and the learner has learnt	
Step 4	Group reflection on the teaching	Pendleton's rules of the consultation

To help others to use our ideas we have included an example of this method after the descriptions of step 1 and step 2.

Step 1 "creating the learning need".

Wlodkowski (Wlodkowski R J 1985) speaks tellingly of "creating the right degree of discomfort"- enough to motivate learning, but not so much as to paralyse. Learning should not be painless, but "worthy of the discomfort required". Knowles (Knowles M 1987) was clear that adult learners had to be convinced of the value of an educational experience in the light of their self-concept as an autonomous person, and of the developmental needs of their social roles.

Example of step 1

The participants are presented with the following table of results (which is a simplified version of the results of the 4S trial);

Table 2

	Dead	Alive	Total
Placebo	5	95	100
Statin	3	97	100

They are then split into two groups to argue for and against statin treatment according to tabloid headlines. One group is told that they are journalists and that the proprietor of their tabloid has just bought a company making statins. They must write headlines which persuade their readers to buy them. The other group work are journalists working for the rival paper and must rubbish statins.

Step 2 - transmitting knowledge.
This is the traditional step of transmitting knowledge and it is in this step that the new concepts are taught. While the first step can often be usefully structured as group work (though it may be a story or something else) the second step is best structured in something like lecture format. This is because, following Professor Elton from the Institute of Education, groups are good at changing attitudes but lectures are a good way to transmit knowledge. In this step computational methods may or may not be used.

Example of step 2

When the futility of arguing in headlines has sunk in they are taken slowly through the definitions of the various statistics used in therapeutic trials, using the numbers from the example above.

Balloons and Teddy bears

A distinction is drawn between statistics which are invariant, and those that depend on the frequency of the event in the population in question. Invariant statistics such as RRR are large, and hence the favourite of drug reps and scientists. A large, suitably labelled Teddy bear can be introduced to reinforce this point. Statistics that vary, depending on the underlying population rate, such as ARR and NNT, are more meaningful to patients and clinicians. They can be illustrated by a balloon.

Event rate in control group

C.E.R. =

Event rate in experimental group

E.E.R. =

Actual Risk Reduction

A.R.R. = (C.E.R. - E.E.R.)

A.R.R. =

Relative Risk Reduction

R.R.R. = A.R.R. / C.E.R.

R.R.R. =

Number needed to treat

N.N.T. = 1/A.R.R.

N.N.T. =

Step 3 - checking.

Step 3 is to check that the teacher knows that he has taught and the learner that he has learnt. It can be done in a wide variety of ways; by repeating the development of the concept with a different worked example, by giving out worksheets, etc...

Step 4 - feedback.

This is the step where the student moves from learning to learning how to teach. It is analogous to Pendleton's rules for the consultation, this is a vital ten minutes at the end of the teaching session when all participants feed-back on the quality of the teaching, going round the circle giving positive comments about what was helpful, then ideas about what might have gone better. Finally, you check that everybody is feeling comfortable. This step is important for the teacher so that he can continually improve his teaching.

It is important for the learners because it enables them to feedback tactfully where they have lost the thread. It is also part of the attraction of the method that doctors are much more willing to learn how to teach statistics (which sounds and indeed is important) than to learn statistics (which they feel they should already know and have already learnt and forgotten many times before).

Relationship to other attempts to teach statistics.

One of the bestselling books on statistics is called "Statistics without tears" by Rowntree (Rowntree 1981). He distinguishes between computational methods for users and non-computational methods for consumers. A non-computational method is a story, group exercise or any other method that does not involve working with numbers. In our model step 1 is non-computational though step 2 may have a computational element. He talks about statistics without tears but not without effort, and similarly we try to avoid frightening people, but certainly encourage them to work at understanding, for example by knowing they will have to teach.

The charismatic John Allen Paulos (John Allen Paulos 1996) wrote a successful book about teaching mathematics by means of stories. Knowledge of statistics is traditionally seen as hierarchical, that is, that each new step depends on understanding all the previous ones. In contrast he points out that there is, in practice, little difficulty in carving out small chunks of statistics which can be taught in isolation.

Evidence for effectiveness

The strength of the four step method, having run it now in some five very varied groups, is that people do learn, and in an enjoyable way. Moreover, stories have a mnemonic power that numbers will never match. In one group of students who received a pre and post course questionnaire there was a significant increase in their score for confidence in understanding and willingness to teach both the statistics taught and statistics in general.

It does, however, have an obvious weakness. It is slow. It takes a good half hour to get one set of related concepts across. It is, however, perhaps better to "teach less so that we can learn more".

Conclusion

Doctors need mathematical skills. We describe a method for teaching groups of doctors who do not feel confident about their mathematical skills. While traditional methods leave some students feeling crushed, we have found that this method empowers student and leaves them keen and able to pass on their new knowledge.

References

John Allen Paulos 1996, *A mathematician reads the newspaper* Penguin, London.

Knowles M 1987, "Androgogy: an emerging technology for adult learning," in *Adult learning and education*, Tight M, ed., Oxford University Press, Oxford, pp. 53-70.

Rowntree 1981, *Statistics without tears* Penguin books, London.

Wlodkowski R J 1985, "Integrating emotions with learning," in *Enhancing adult motivation to learn*, Jossey Bass, pp. 178-212.

In the following short article a point, made in the previous article, is elaborated for a different audience.

Teaching tip: balloons and teddy bears
Evid Based Med 2006;**11**:39 doi:10.1136/ebm.11.2.39

We all know that the choice of the measure of effect (RRR, ARR, or NNT) influences attitudes to a treatment. But how do we make this memorable for students? There are two types of "statistics": those whose value does depend on the underlying frequency of a disease and those statistics whose value does depend not on it ("invariant statistics"). Thus, RRR and its friends RBI and RRI are invariant statistics. Their value does not alter depending on the underlying incidence of the condition in the population described. On the other hand, NNT (and ARR) have values that do depend on this. Typically, NNT will be very large for a rare condition (because many people have to be treated to reach one person with the condition), while it will be smaller in a population where this disease is commoner. This distinction applies to diagnosis also, e.g., likelihood ratios are invariant whereas predictive values depend on the prevalence or pre-test probability.

The two types of measurements can be brought home by bringing to the teaching session two unusual ingredients: a large teddy bear and a balloon. At an appropriate point the teddy, which will have already caught the attention of the learners, can be cuddled as the lecturer explains that RRRs are beloved of two groups of people, scientists and drug reps. Scientists love them because they are invariant and thus only need to be calculated once. Drug reps love them because they are large (for example a 50% reduction in risk) and can therefore help to sell products, even where this is inappropriate because in a particular population the condition is rare and therefore the actual risk reduction (ARR) is small. This can be illustrated by some suitable study such as the use of statins in groups with a low and high incidence of ischaemic heart disease.

NNTs on the other hand are useful to doctors and patients. This is because they tell the doctor what the benefit is to the patient of the treatment in question. While explaining this balloon can be inflated, with the letters NNT already written on to it, so that the variable size can be emphasized. I have used this teaching aid with groups of health workers of varying degrees of experience of EBM, and it seems make memorable entities (RRR, NNT) which might otherwise remain boring statistics.

Before the advent of the "Evidence based medicine" movement, I had been, like many general practitioners of my generation, responsible for the computerisation of our practice. In one of the more amusing incidents, a previous practice manager hid the first system we bought in a cupboard, thus delaying its introduction by some months.

The following article was published before the MSc. and helped me gain a place on it. The method (method 2) described is now widely used in computer system, though not as widely and systematically as I had hoped at the time. It is, to my knowledge, the first published description of this method.

Ensuring the accuracy and completeness of clinical data on general practice systems
Journal of Informatics in Primary Care   November 1998

Introduction
Ensuring the accuracy and completeness of clinical data on general practice systems is clearly crucial. The value of the whole enterprise is dependent on the quality of the data. What little published work there is suggests that the quality even in committed

practices leaves something to be desired 1.2. The situation with many hospital systems is probably worse. I wish to share two simple and effective methods for continuously improving the quality of the data.

Methods

Method 1

Most of the numeric data is more or less normally distributed unlike the errors in the data which will tend to a random distribution. Therefore, the data at either end of the distribution will be that most likely to be inaccurate. It can be extracted and checked manually.

An example is blood pressure. The highest and lowest values will contain a lot of data entry errors. Another example is any distribution against age. The youngest people in any data set who appear to have a certain condition have a fair chance of not having it in reality. The youngest person in our surgery with a recording of pernicious anaemia turned out on inspection of hospital letters to have been proven *not* to have it. We were unable to persuade her to stop her three monthly injections, but that is another story.

Method 2

This is illustrated by *Table 1,* overleaf.

The basic idea is that there are certain classes of drugs that imply a specific diagnosis or diagnoses. In Table 1 the figures are for drugs of each class ever prescribed during the previous eight years (since the computer system was introduced). The number of "correct" diagnoses entered almost never reaches 100% because of (a) rarer indications, and (b) data entry errors. However, trawling through the notes of those with a drug without an appropriate diagnosis will reveal some data entry omissions. This can be an iterative process. The table records the results of two consecutive trawls two years apart. The second trawl included a branch surgery not covered the first time. Nevertheless, the results emphasize that data quality will deteriorate without constant vigilance. In the case of our general practice we have on average a 10% yearly turnover of patients.

The data extraction process could be significantly automated using MIQUEST and run yearly to maintain data quality.

Drug	Disease	1996	1998
		% with diagnosis	% with diagnosis
ACE inhibitors	Hypertension, CCF	93%	93%
Bendrofluazide 2.5mg	Hypertension	86%	86%
Calcium antagonists	Hypertension, Angina, Raynaud's	91%	95%
Nitrates	Angina	77%	86%
Digoxin	AF	62%	67%
SSRIs	Anxiety/depression	84%	88%
Some anti-epileptics	Epilepsy	70%	70%
Asthma "preventers"	Asthma/COPD	89%	94%
Diabetic drugs	Diabetes	92%	98%
Thyroxine	Hypothyroidism, Ca thyroid	91%	94%
Anti-thyroid drugs	Hyperthyroidism	71%	100%
Drugs for glaucoma	Glaucoma	92%	87%
Beta-blockers	Hypertension,		85%

	anxiety, migraine		
Allopurinol	Gout	82%	94%
Anti-parkinsonian drugs	Parkinson's	83&	76%
Hydroxycobalamin	Non-Fe def, anaemia	76%	71%
Tamoxifen	Ca breast	82%	87%

References

1 Whitelaw FG, Taylor RJ, Nevin SL Taylor MW, Milne RM, Watt AH. Completeness and accuracy of morbidity and repeat prescribing records held on general practice computers in Scotland. *Br* J Gen *Pract* 1996; 46:181-186

2 Pringle M. Ward p, Chilvers C. Assessment of the completeness and accuracy of computer medical records in four practices committed to recording data on computer. *Br* J Gen *Pract* 1995; 45:537-541

Articles about refugees and asylum seekers

After the MSc I looked for some part time academic work, but found no opening. I applied to become the course organiser for our local VTS (vocational training scheme) but was not chosen; they suggested that, having worked with VSO, I should work with refugees. Eventually I worked part time as a medical report writer at what was then called; "The Medical Foundation for the care of survivors of torture, now "Freedom from torture". It was work that needed to be done and which, as the son of my mother who had been a refugee, I found that I could do. My wife, though, told me it that took its toll on me. It was a privilege to meet many brave people most of whom believed that settled status in the UK was essential to their survival. I can remember, among others, an Eritrean who had endured imprisonment in a military camp in the desert simply for preaching the Gospel. Beyond the medico-legal work, important as that was, there was another dimension. It was a question of reaching out and touching another person. Often the message was; "you are a good person, you are a person to whom bad things have happened; you are not a bad person"[6]. While working at the Medical Foundation I met Dr Rayah Feldman, an academic sociologist. Together we wrote a standard introduction to primary care for refugees that we updated from time to time and which was something of a centrepiece for the website on refugee care hosted by the Department of Health. One fine day, however, the Department, doubtless for political reasons, took down its refugee care website together with our review. Despite assurances that they would reappear they were never seen again, a lesson in

---

[6] This is very similar to the words Sirius Black says to console Harry Potter in "The order of the Phoenix"; "You're not a bad person. You're a very good person, who bad things have happened to." Voldermort has been entering Harry's mind in order to make Harry think he is an evil person like Voldermort. In the same way torturers, often systematically, by lies, insults, rape and other torture, attempt to make their victims think they are bad people. Of more relevance to mainstream general practice, the same occurs in cases of abuse of all sorts.

the transitoriness of resources hosted on the web. A version had however been stored at another site[7]. Our material, updated yet again, found its last home as the chapter of a book[8].

The situation of refugees, both legal and social, changes rapidly in the UK. Details, in the articles below, correct at the time of writing will since have changed.

The pieces include a number of campaigning articles for the BJGP, an article about teaching primary care for refugees and a talk to the girls at Chelmsford High school.

Government proposes to end free health care for "failed asylum seekers"

Br J Gen Pract. 2006 Jan 1; 56(522): 59.

We wish to warn GPs about the current proposals to make "failed asylum seekers" ineligible for free primary care. The government defines a failed asylum seeker as a person whose asylum application has been refused and who is deemed to have exhausted all available channels for appeal. However, those who are unsuccessful at appeal are not necessarily here illegally. For example they may be awaiting an outcome of a further legal challenge or cannot return to their country of origin due to the human rights situation there (1) (2). They include those who have yet to be returned. Often "failed asylum seekers" have simply been unable to prove that they would suffer persecution if returned (3). The Cambridge Institute of Criminology has described the culture at the home office as "a culture of disbelief" (4) and organisations such as the Medical Foundation for the Victims of Torture and Amnesty International have criticised the poor quality of initial asylum decisions (5).

---

[7] http://repository.forcedmigration.org/pdf/?pid=fmo:5929

[8] Vernon G, Feldman R. Refugees and asylum seekers in primary care; from looking after to working together. In: Gill PS, Wright N, Brew I, editors. Working with Vulnerable Groups: A Clinical Handbook for GPs. London: RCGP; 2014.

Nevertheless, it is from this group of failed asylum seekers that the government is trying to remove entitlement to free primary care (6) (7). They would remain eligible to emergency and immediately necessary treatment and the treatment of certain infectious diseases, notably not including HIV/AIDS.

Under the guise of concern to limit health expenditure the present government appears to be trying to limit provision for "failed asylum seekers" for political ends. Since April 2004 "failed asylum seekers" are entitled to secondary care only at the discretion of the hospital. Since last year the government has been considering a proposal to make "failed asylum seekers" ineligible for free primary care (7-9). This proposal is an example of the "Fortress Europe" mentality, widespread throughout Europe, which restricts the access of migrant workers to health care (10) (11).

It is both ethically wrong and unworkable. It is ethically wrong because the most destitute group in the country, who cannot legally work, is being denied a basic service. It is unworkable because general practices do not have the skills or resources to carry out immigration checks to identify the small number of "failed asylum seekers" among the large pool of other foreign born patients, nor are such checks part of their health care remit. Restricting access to this group also increases the risk to public health if cases of TB and HIV are left unidentified and untreated. On all these grounds this policy has been roundly condemned by the House of Commons Health Select Committee (12).

Such regulations would further confuse those health professionals who already, wrongly, believe that asylum seekers are not entitled to primary care, as well as refugees and asylum seekers themselves who might avoid seeking necessary healthcare whatever their entitlement. Providing free primary care services for all asylum seekers is the only way to ensure both individual welfare and public health.

Reference List

(1) IPPR. Migration and health in the UK. London: IPPR
http://www.ippr.org.uk/ecomm/files/migration_health_factf
ile.pdf (accessed 18/09/05); 2005.

(2) Manavi K, Welsby PD. HIV testing. BMJ 2005 Mar
5;330(7490):492-3.

(3) Williams P. Why failed asylum seekers must not be denied
access to the NHS. BMJ 2004 Jul 31;329:298.

(4) Webber L, Gelsthorpe L. Deciding to detain: How
decisions to detain asylum seekers are made at ports of
entry. Cambridge: Institute of Criminology, University of
Cambridge; 2000.

(5) Ward K, Henson R. Decision making and appeals process.
2005. London, ICAR. ICAR Statistics paper 2.
Ref Type: Generic

(6) Ashcroft R. Standing up for the medical rights of asylum
seekers. J Med Ethics 2005;31:125-6.

(7) Department of Health. Proposals to Exclude Overseas
Visitors from Eligibility to Free NHS Primary Medical
Services; A Consultation. London: Department of Health
http://www.dh.gov.uk/Consultations/ClosedConsultations/
ClosedConsultationsArticle/fs/en?CONTENT_ID=408761
8&chk=YG1MPh (accessed 18/09/2005); 2004.

(8) Department of Health. Table of entitlement to NHS
treatment (Correct as of January 2005). London:
Department of Health
http://www.dh.gov.uk/PolicyAndGuidance/International/As
ylumSeekersAndRefugees/fs/en (accessed 18/09/2005);
2005.

(9)   Department of Health. Hutton proposes tighter NHS rules for treating overseas visitors. London: Department of Health www.dh.gov.uk/PublicationsAndStatistics/PressReleases/PressReleasesNotices/fs/en%3FCONTENT_ID%3D4047476%26chk%3DAbL%252BD9 (accessed 18/09/2005); 2005.

(10)   Romero-Ortuno R. Access to health care for illegal immigrants in the EU: should we be concerned. European Journal of Health Law 2004;11:245-72.

(11)   Norredam M, Mygind A, Krasnik A. Access to health care for asylum seekers in the European Union - a comparative study of country policies. European Journal of public Health 2005 Oct 17.

(12)   House of Commons Health Select Committee. New Developments in HIV/AIDS and Sexual Health Policy. London: Houses of Parliament http://www.publications.parliament.uk/pa/cm200405/cmselect/cmhealth/252/25202.htm (accessed 18/09/2005); 2005.

An Alarm Bell

BJGP 58 (549): 285-285; 2008.

I wish to ring an alarm bell. The facts may not be unfamiliar to general practitioners who work in particular inner-city areas, but may be quite new to GPs who live and work in "middle England". Many mornings somewhere in the UK a private security van sets out. It belongs to a company sub-contracted by the Home Office. It will arrive at its destination in the early morning, while the family is still asleep. They will be woken by a loud knock and given half an hour to pack their bags. Children will be woken too and given the same instructions. They will be taken to a detention centre. On other occasions similar vans have picked up teenage children while they wait at the school bus stop. In some cases where a child fails to attend school, this has been the reason.

These families are not criminals, some are in the process of applying for asylum, others have finished the process; the group which the home office calls "failed asylum seekers". However many "failed asylum seekers" have failed in their asylum application not because their claim was unjust, but because of the Home Office's "culture of disbelief" (1). An employee of one of these security firms told me he had taken the job because no qualifications were required. Some of his colleagues have an army or police background. Do they never beat up their clients when they fail to co-operate, scream or become hysterical (2)? They will be taken to a detention centre from which many will be returned to their home countries. Here some will be arrested again, some tortured and some will be at risk of being killed.

As a society we are training up a group of people to whom this is their daily work. They tend to pick on families who are isolated, have perhaps been here for a while and are not in the middle of their own communities where a riot might be sparked.

As well as the security officers we are training a vast tribe of bureaucrats at the Home Office to whom all this is ordinary paperwork.

Today they are coming for the asylum seekers, to-morrow who will they come for?

Much of this information I have heard first hand from clients at the "Medical Foundation for the Care of Victims of Torture," (http://www.torturecare.org.uk/) some from other GPs working with asylum seekers and refugees. Harm during deportation has been documented by the "Medical Foundation" (2). News reports scattered in the media are collected by the Institute of Race Relations; http://www.irr.org.uk/. A recent book by a member of the Institute gives a more exhaustive account of this process of removal with extensive references (3).

Much can be done. Doctors who wish to help clients in detention centres may contact an organisation called "Medical Justice" http://www.medicaljustice.org.uk/ which seeks to improve health care during immigration detention. Those who believe a limited amnesty may help can contact "Strangers into Citizens" http://www.strangersintocitizens.org.uk/. For the first time since the beginning of the Second World War substantial numbers of people resident in the UK no longer have access to free primary care. This number may suddenly increase substantially if the Department of Health's current review, due to report in December, decides that "failed asylum seekers" should no longer have access to free primary care (4). A last ditch campaign to prevent this is being run by "Medact"; http://www.medact.org/article_refugee.php?articleID=691. As a result, we are seeing the return of charitable organisations offering free primary care. There are two in London; "Médecins Sans Frontières"

 http://www.msf.org/unitedkingdom/index.cfm and "Médecins du Monde" http://www.medecinsdumonde.org.uk/projectlondon/default.asp, both of them are looking for volunteer GPs.

Reference List

(1) Webster L, Gelsthorpe L. Deciding to detain: How decisions to detain asylum seekers are made at ports of entry. Cambridge: Institute of Criminology; 2000.

(2) Granville-Chapman C, Smith E, Moloney M. Harm on removal: excessive force against failed asylum seekers. London: Medical Foundation for the Care of Victims of Torture; 2004.

(3) Kundani A. Here to stay. The end of Tolerance. London: Pluto Press; 2007. p. 153-64.

(4) Vernon G, Feldman R. Government proposes to end free health care for "failed asylum seekers". BJGP 2006 Jan;56(522):59.

"Home office syndrome" (2008)

Br J Gen Pract. 2008 Jul;58(552):510

The Editor,

Br J Gen Pract.

Dear Sir,

We wish to offer a name for a syndrome which will be familiar to those working with refugees and asylum seekers. While asylum seekers are awaiting a Home Office decision on their asylum claim they often give no attention to their other needs and in particular their health needs. This is because they often fear that they will be killed or tortured if they are returned to the countries from which they came.

Asylum seeker patients' health and health behaviour is strongly influenced by their social circumstances - starting with the events that have happened in the countries they have come from, the stress of separation from their family and everything that is familiar, and the difficulties they face here. Once in the UK, taking care of their health, or bothering to take tablets for conditions such as high blood pressure or diabetes seems unimportant compared to the immediate problems of survival. Health problems take second place to the progress of their asylum case - people will miss important appointments with their GP or hospital specialist to see their solicitor.

The "Home Office syndrome" is perhaps a specific example of Maslow's hierarchy of needs. While the individual is dealing with what he perceives to be a threat to his life all other matters including healthcare are put on hold.

The delays in deciding asylum status have been long and may still last months. As a result, the "Home Office syndrome" is bad for the health of asylum seekers who may wait long periods before they seek appropriate help for their health needs. Other examples of policies which damage the health of asylum seekers are those which prevent legal employment (1), and the refusal of secondary health care for "failed" asylum seekers. The last policy has recently been judged illegal in the High Court (2),

Yours Sincerely,

Dr Gervase Vernon, GP and medico-legal report writer,

Medical Foundation for the care of victims of torture, London N7 7JW

Dave Ridley, Practice Nurse

Cape Hill Medical Centre, Smethwick, West Midlands

Dineo Lesetedi, Practice Nurse,

The Meridian Practice, Coventry

Reference List

(1) Vernon G, Feldman R. Refugees in Primary Care: from looking after to working together. http://www networks nhs uk/uploads/06/06/refugees_in_primary_care doc 2006Available from: URL: http://www.networks.nhs.uk/uploads/06/06/refugees_in_primary_care.doc

(2) DoH. Failed asylum seekers and ordinary residence. DoH 2008 May 11Available from: URL: http://www.dh.gov.uk/en/Publicationsandstatistics/Lettersandcirculars/Dearcolleagueletters/DH_084479

I was a trainer in general practice for many years, having re-introduced training to the practice after a lapse of some years. I much enjoyed it and only stopped because I could no longer cope with the ever increasing paper work. I also presented various papers at local and regional trainers' workshops in the days before these became solely concerned with administrative matters. The paper which follows first was presented at the annual East Anglia trainers' workshop.

How to teach trainees about primary care for refugees and asylum speakers

Vernon, G. How to teach trainees about primary care for refugees and asylum seekers. Education for primary care 2008;19(4):430-2.

In each vocational training scheme area there is likely to be at least one practice that has a substantial population of refugees or asylum seekers. These practices have built up ways of dealing with these patients which should be shared with other practices in the VTS. Even if our own practice has few such patients, refugees and asylum seekers are a group with whom our trainees are quite likely to work at some time during their career. It is therefore our responsibility to make such training available to them. Moreover, treating people from other cultures makes explicit what is equally true for people from our own culture: that each individual has different ideas about illness and different expectations about doctors. Treating refugees, then, can force trainees to ask explicitly about the patients' health beliefs. This can be more difficult with UK born patients where the trainee may naively and quite wrongly assume that the patient in front of him shares his beliefs and expectations.

Such teaching can be achieved in different ways. It can be delivered in a suitable practice, if it has many refugees. Trainees can gain experience by swapping practices. Finally, it can be delivered at the VTS. Many vocational training schemes will have trainees who have experienced forced migration. While they may be a useful resource, their sensitivities should be taken into account during such training.

The teaching that is to be offered can, as is conventional, be divided into knowledge, skills and attitudes.

Knowledge
There are many different sorts of migrants in the UK; legal migrants and their dependants (about 2.8 million), illegal migrants, on whom the catering and hospitality industry of the South-East depends (about ½ million), settled refugees (maybe ¼ million) and "failed asylum seekers" (at least 100,000). "Failed asylum seekers" are asylum seekers who have not been accepted by the Home Office as refugees under the Geneva Convention and who have exhausted all legal avenues in the UK. Some, however, cannot be removed from the UK as they come from a failed state, for example Somalia. As well as knowledge about refugee types, it is necessary to have some knowledge about the legal framework and about access to NHS treatment.

 Knowledge, as usual, is the easiest thing to teach and a lecture format is quite appropriate. There are good articles by Burnett and Peel (1) (2) (3). There is an excellent internet site;

http://www.networks.nhs.uk/networks.php?pid=256

It contains a simple bibliography and the proceedings of the second national conference on this topic which includes several excellent power point presentations. Finally, that site contains a detailed review article written by myself and Dr Rayah Feldman which we attempt to keep up to date.

http://www.networks.nhs.uk/uploads/06/06/refugees_in_primary_care.doc

Once knowledge has been assimilated, it can be tested on an internet tutorial on doctors.net. It is necessary to register with doctors.net; but there is no charge. You do not need the exact address; simply log on to doctors.net and search for the tutorial about asylum seekers.

http://www.doctors.net.uk/ecme/wfrmmcq.aspx?testtype=pre&gro
upid=43&moduleid=476&orgnid=3

Skills

There are a number of specific skills required. The one most
widely applicable is the use of interpreters. Family interpreters are
acceptable for simple matters. PCTs have a duty to provide
interpreting services, though some choose to do so via a telephone
link (language line; http://www.languageline.com/). The doctor
must learn to speak in simple but complete sentences, avoiding
medical jargon, enabling the interpreter to deal with one coherent
chunk at a time. When the patient answers it is important to look at
their body language, not at the interpreter. It is a good idea to greet
the interpreter by name and generally make them feel a valued
member of the team. Knowing a few words of the language,
especially if it is one common in your practice area, will enhance
your standing with both the patient and the interpreter.

Most of our registrars speak more than one language, so that a role
play amongst the trainees is a form of training that could usefully
follow a short didactic session. A PCT interpreter might be
persuaded to attend. There are more details on interpreting in the
review referenced above. Other skills which might be taught, also
referenced in that review, would be dealing with victims of rape or
torture.

However, one question which trainees will often raise is how to
contain the consultation; how to deal with many apparently
insoluble problems in a ten minute consultation. There is a useful
power point presentation by Dr Pugh on this topic which can be
downloaded free. Again, the issues are not specific to refuges but
would resonate with many of our consultations.

http://www.networks.nhs.uk/uploads/06/03/refugeeconf/pugh.ppt

Attitudes

The hardest thing to teach can be to get registrar to understand
"what it feels like to be a refugee." A powerful technique in the

one to one setting is to get the trainee to choose some part of their life when they may have experienced something similar; an experience of migration, or going to boarding school as a small child. As they talk about it the penny may drop that the overwhelming feelings that assailed them then is what the refugee patient is experiencing now. In the VTS group situation this would be an opportunity to use a suitable film clip or other material. I have found Auden's poem "Refugee Blues" effective in many different groups, typically producing a stunned silence. An excellent course for medical undergraduates dealing survivors of violence and conflicts in the community has been described in this journal (4).

To summarise; teaching our trainees how to deal with patients who are refugees and asylum seekers can be done. It should be done because this is something our trainees may well have to do wherever they end up. The skills they will learn are mostly those that are basic to all general practice; the hard practical work of finding out how somebody else thinks and feels.

Reference List

(1)   Burnett A, Peel M. Asylum seekers and refugees in Britain: The health of survivors of torture and organised violence. BMJ 2001;322:606-9.

(2)   Burnett A, Peel M. Asylum seekers and refugees in Britain: What brings asylum seekers to the United Kingdom? BMJ 2001;322:485-8.

(3)   Burnett A, Peel M. Asylum seekers and refugees in Britain: Health needs of asylum seekers and refugees. BMJ 2001;322:544-7.

(4)   Osonnaya C, Osonnaya K, Sanderson I. Effects of conflicts,
       violence and torture in the community: a challenge for
       primary and community care teachers. Education for
       primary care 2005;16(312-316).

*The following article is a report on a Europe wide conference on
refugee matters hosted by the JRS Europe (the Jesuit Refuge
Service) in Brussels.*

Denunciation; a new threat to access to health care for undocumented migrants
Br J Gen Pract. 2012 Feb; 62(595): 98–99.

In February of this year I went to a European meeting on the care
of undocumented migrants (JRS Europe 2011). There are
estimated to be 2.6 to 6.4 million across the European Union (1/2
% to 1% of the population of the EU) (IOM 2008) and half a
million such undocumented migrants in the UK . The hospitality
industry in the South-East of England depends heavily on them, so
that one person's illegal immigrant is another person's helpful
waiter (Vernon and Feldman 2006). As the conference was running
thousands were landing on the Italian island of Lampedusa to
avoid the Libyan crisis. I will first review what is already
established about access to health care for undocumented migrants,
then describe a new threat highlighted at this conference;
denunciation.

The current situation regarding the health care of legal migrants in
the EU has been well described by two officials from the
International Organisation for Migration (IOM); "European
countries face a threefold situation of: (i) constant migrant flows,
(ii) health services and practices that are largely inaccessible or
unused by migrant populations and often ill-suited to migrants'
needs and (iii) higher vulnerability of migrants and their children
to ill health due to negative socioeconomic circumstances. On the
other hand, protection of migrants' health and their access to
quality health care are recognised as: (i) a human right and a basic
entitlement according to EU values; (ii) vital to migrants'

integration and critical to reduce poverty and (iii) essential for social cohesion, good public health and the wellbeing of all (Peiro and Benedict 2010)." Where the migrant is legal the EU is committed to improving access to health care. In contrast where the migrant is undocumented or illegal the health practitioner is placed in a dilemma; on the one hand, if they wish to provide care, they may be breaking legal or financial regulations, on the other hand, if they do not provide care, they may be violating human rights laws and acting against their own conscience (Karl-Trummer et al. 2010).

There were many themes to the conference and one was certainly the great variety of responses to the situation from different European states. It was sobering to learn that the in the UK undocumented migrants have less rights for access to health care than in the Netherlands, France, Spain or Portugal (Karl-Trummer, Novak-Zezulqa, & Metzler 2010). Yet for undocumented child migrants this right is enshrined in the legally binding "United Nations Convention on the Rights of the Child" (1989) an international treaty signed by all members of the United Nations, including the UK, excepting only Somalia and the USA (United Nations 2011).Yearly reports have found the UK in breach of the Convention. (The rights of migrants, legal and undocumented, to health have been summarized by the International Organization for Migration (IOM) (Pace 2010). A recent EU conference has re-affirmed these rights (8th Conference of European Health Ministers 2007)).Some states, France and Italy for example, provide specialised and anonymous access to health care for undocumented migrants (HUMA network 2009) (Karl-Trummer, Novak-Zezulqa, & Metzler 2010). (The situation with regard to access to health care across Europe is monitored by PICUM's newsletters and its academic collaboration; "MIGHEALTHNET" (PICUM (Platform for International Co-operation on Undocumented Migrants) 2011))

Availability of health care in different EU states depends on the legislative context. States with an insurance-based health system can differentiate between legal access and funding, often providing one and not the other, whereas these two are conflated in tax-based systems. Beyond the legislative context is the everyday practice. Some countries may provide better access in reality in spite of a restrictive legislative context. This is often because of the activity of NGOs working on behalf of migrant communities. Such NGOs have sprung up in many countries; two active in the UK today are "Médecins du Monde" and "Médecins sans Frontières." In the UK some migrants may access health care either on an emergency basis, which is legal, or via registration with a general practitioner (which is only legal in the case of asylum seekers and failed asylum seekers (RCGP 2011).) In the UK the criterion for access to health care is residence. Before 2004 this could be taken to include undocumented migrants, but in that year the House of Lords refined the concept of residence to mean lawful residence, specifically excluding undocumented migrants.

There are some trends across European states of which UK doctors should be aware. The most widespread is the denial of health care as an instrument of immigration policy. This is occurring in every state. To some extent it is co-ordinated at a European level because there is a central European policy on immigration; sometimes called "Fortress Europe" by its denigrators. In contrast health care provision is largely devolved to the member states. This use of the denial of heath care as an instrument of immigration policy is, in my view, both manifestly unjust and ineffective. Do the policy makers really think that potential economic migrants research current health provision in the member state before migrating? This policy also has negative public health consequences as ill people are delayed in accessing health care and may therefore pose a risk to public health((HUMA network 2009) p.179).

The new trend highlighted at the conference was denunciation. Denunciation is where a state makes it a duty, or a condition of employment, for certain citizens to report undocumented migrants to the authorities. In the UK this has been a creeping trend over the past decades, so that now government employees in housing departments, benefit offices and schools have such a duty (Cohen 2006). In hospitals this does not fall to hospital doctors, but special people called "overseas payment officers." These employees simply have a duty to assess whether a patient can be charged, not, so far as I know, to denounce to the immigration authorities. Some however may do so. There was a pilot at the Central Middlesex Hospital near Heathrow where a direct line was installed between the hospital and the immigration service for the purpose of establishing immigration status. At Milton Keynes hospital, ward clerks are given a clear duty to report any suspicion that a patient is not a UK resident to the overseas payment officer. This officer's primary role is clearly to recover money. Appendix 8 of the hospital overseas payments policy, however, is a form that the overseas payment officer may use to fax a query to the immigration authorities in order to verify a patient's status. This form, while not being mandatory, will clearly, if used, act as a form of denunciation to the immigration authorities (Milton Keynes Hospital 2009). Whatever the precise situation, fear of being denounced and then deported is a frequently cited barrier for access to health care ((Medecins du Monde 2009) p. 93.)

Perhaps because GPs in the UK are self-employed it has not been suggested that they denounce patients to the authorities. However in Italy a law making it a duty for all doctors to denounce undocumented migrants seeking treatment was passed in the Chamber of Deputies by the Berlusconi government in 2009 (Medecins du Monde 2009). Because the various Italian doctors' unions co-operated for once and threatened to go on strike this law was defeated in the Senate. In Germany entitlement to care for undocumented migrants is effectively barred by the obligation to denounce imposed by German legislation on public institutions including the social welfare centres that have competencies on public health issues ((HUMA network 2009) p.15).

A further threat, not as yet enshrined in any European law, as far as I am aware, is criminalisation. Criminalisation is where helping undocumented migrant in a specified way – such as providing health care – is made a criminal offence. However, many years ago in Pinochet's Chile it was illegal to treat opponents of the regime. A British doctor, Sheila Cassidy was imprisoned and tortured for this offence. She wrote a moving account of this (Cassidy 1992). Similar action is being taken today in Bahrain against doctors who helped protestors in the "Arab Spring" pro-democracy demonstration.

Denunciation as a basis of public policy is very corrosive of trust. It has been depicted in a recent episode of Coronation Street, and perhaps more memorably by Arthur Miller in "A view from the bridge" (Miller 1955).The sad truth is that most of us can denounce somebody in a moment of spite and regret the action once it is too late.

I hope this piece may serve as a warning to UK doctors to look at the situation beyond our own borders and resolve not to be led down the two dangerous paths of denunciation and criminalisation, but to support policies that enable access to health care by all migrants. Migration is an increasing phenomenon in our modern world and migrants can bring great benefits to the host society if they are properly integrated.

References

8th Conference of European Health Ministers. Bratislava declaration on health human rights and migration. 2007. Ref Type: Bill/Resolution

Cassidy, S. 1992. *Audacity to believe* London, Datman Longman and Todd.

Cohen, S. 2006. *Deportation is Freedom!: The Orwellian World of Immigration Controls* Lolndon, Jessica Kingsley Publishers.

HUMA network 2009, *Accesss to health care for undocumented migrants and asylum seekers in 10 EU countries*, HUMA network.

IOM 2008, *2008 World Migration Report*, International Organisation for Migration, Geneva.

JRS Europe Invisible borders; migrant destitution in Europe; Brussels March 2011, Brussels.

Karl-Trummer, U., Novak-Zezulqa, S., & Metzler, B. 2010. Acces to health care for undocumented migrants in the EU: a first lanscape of NowHereLand. *Eurohealth*, 16, (1) 13-16

Medecins du Monde 2009, *Accesss to health care for undocumented migrants in 11 EU countries*, Medecins du Monde.

Miller, A. 1955. *A view from the bridge* London, Penguin Modern Classics 2010.

Milton Keynes Hospital. Milton Keynes Hospital overseas patients' policy. 1-9-2009.
Ref Type: Online Source

Pace, P. 2010. What can be done in EU member states to protect the health of migrants? *Eurohealth*, 16, (1) 5-10

Peiro, M. & Benedict, R. 2010. Migrant health policy, the Portuguese and Spanish EU presidencies. *Eurohealth*, 16, (1) 4

PICUM (Platform for International Co-operation on Undocumented Migrants). MIGHEALTHNET.
http://mighealth.net/uk/index.php/Refugees_and_asylum_seekers_-_Accessibility_of_care accessed 21/05/2011 . 2011.
Ref Type: Electronic Citation

RCGP. Failed Asylum Seekers / Vulnerable Migrants and Access to Primary Care. RCGP . 2011.
Ref Type: Electronic Citation

United Nations. United Nations Convention on the Rights of the Child (1989). 2011.
Ref Type: Online Source

Vernon, G. & Feldman, R. Refugees in Primary Care: from looking after to working together.
http://repository.forcedmigration.org/pdf/?pid=fmo:5934 accessed 12/05/2011 . 2006.
Ref Type: Electronic Citation

Talk on refugees and asylum seekers Chelmsford High School (2014)

How does it feel to be a refugee?

Perhaps the following analogy will help. Do you remember your first day at a new school? Imagine that the other students are speaking a foreign language, though one you can understand.

Everything is new and you are at the mercy of those already there. Some help you and you remember them for a long time. Others ignore you; yet others go out of their way to be nasty. But refugees cannot go home at the end of the day; they are stuck for good. (Here the Auden poem "Refugee Blues" is shown to the audience).

Why is it of interest to you?

Refugees are currently headline news in the UK, routinely scapegoated in much of the tabloid press. The current crisis is in Syria. Six weeks ago, I wrote to my constituency MP, Sir Alan Hazlehurst, at a time when it seemed unthinkable that the government would accept any refugees from Syria, asking him to allow a few refugees in. I am proud to belong to a nation where I can freely write to my MP. He always replies promptly and courteously, although on this occasion he did reply; "I think that the British public is losing patience with immigration", doubtless reflecting the views of many of his constituents. Today the situation has changed. It seems likely that the government will let in a few refugees; there is a further vote on 29/01/2014 in parliament. My message is "do not give up on what you think is right, because what seemed impossible yesterday, seems difficult the next day and gets done on the third." However, if you too want to influence your own MP it is easy, just Google "Refugee council, Syria" and follow the link. You do not even need to know the name of your MP, it finds it for you.

Rabbi Hugo Gryn was a Holocaust survivor; a survivor of Auschwitz. Today is Holocaust Memorial Day, the 69th anniversary of the liberation of the concentration camp and death factory at Auschwitz. He wrote;

"I believe that future historians will call the twentieth century not only the century of the great wars, but also the century of the refugee. It has been an extraordinary period of movement and upheavals. There are so many scars that need mending and healing and it seems to me that it is imperative that we proclaim that asylum issues are an index of our spiritual and moral civilisation. How you are with the one to whom you owe nothing, that is a grave test and not only as an index of our tragic past. I always think that the real offenders at the half way mark of the century were the bystanders, all those people who let things happen because it didn't affect them directly. I believe that the line our society will take in this matter on how you are to people to whom you owe nothing is a signal. It is the critical signal that we give to our young and I hope and pray that it is a test we shall not fail."In other words; how society deals with refugees sends a signal to other helpless people like our own children.

I would like to give you a little "thought experiment." I have a letter my mother wrote in 1940 to her boyfriend, an English soldier who later became my father, a letter she wrote just before her family had to flee from Italy. In it she complains that her father is insistent that she pack just one suitcase, always kept ready to take with her, because they might have to leave at short notice any day. She signs off the letter writing that she had better get on with this as her father is bound to check up on her. She had to leave behind all her dresses, all her dolls. She took just the one toy, the bear "Boleslaw"; this is him (here my mother's short 6-inch teddy bear is shown to the students). Just imagine quietly for one minute what you would pack in such a bag if you had to flee today.

Why is it of interest to me?

I am a partially retired GP and author. For many years I wrote medico-legal reports for tortured refugees on behalf of a charity;

"Freedom from Torture". My mother was a refugee from Poland and lived on a stateless person's passport in the USA between 1941and 1949. My grandmother was a refugee twice; from the communists in Russia and from Italy in 1940. I wrote her fictionalised biography "Belonging and Betrayal".

Why do people become refugees?

In an area where much research is contentious there is a strong consensus that people become refugees because they are forced by overwhelming circumstances to flee their homes. This is true of my own mother, and of refugees in the UK according to research sponsored by the Home Office (1;2). The origin of asylum seekers in the UK has varied over the last ten years depending on which were the trouble spots in the world at that time. In 2011 they were Pakistan, Iran, Sri Lanka, and Libya. Where they then flee to is a secondary decision often taken by the trafficker.

Here I am talking about refugees; there are also economic migrants but they are in a different category (see below).

The triple trauma of the refugee

Baker has described a triple trauma for refugees;

1) the trauma in their country of origin is so severe that they must flee for their lives,

2) the trauma during forced migration which, due to current regulations, is almost always by illegal means and

3) the trauma of resettlement in the host country (3).

It is the third which is the direct responsibility of the host country and hence of us in the UK. The principal fear of asylum seekers in the UK today is the fear of being detained and deported. The introduction of "fast track" detention has deterred many people from seeking asylum, including, doubtless some genuine refugees. "Fast track" detention means that you are detained on the day you apply and typically until you are deported. Many abuses occur in detention and there is a group that campaigns against these abuses; "Medical Justice".

http://www.medicaljustice.org.uk/

There has been substantial work in Australia by Professor Derek Silove contrasting the mental wellbeing of an earlier phase of Vietnamese refugees who were well accepted by Australian society and the current wave of Middle Eastern refugees who have been largely locked up in camps. Not surprisingly the first group have better mental health and are contributing more to Australian society (4). There is UK evidence that a supportive community can improve the mental health of a refugee who has been tortured (5). This argues against the current UK policy of dispersal which means that refuges cannot settle within their existing communities, but are sent away to an area where they may know nobody.

What is the legal definition of a refugee?

The UN convention on the status of refugees (the 1951 Geneva Convention) defined refugees as "someone who owing to a well-founded fear of being persecuted for reasons of race, religion, nationality, membership of a particular social group or political opinion, is outside the country of his nationality and is unable or, owing to such fear, is unwilling to avail himself of the protection of that country." This replaced the "Nansen passport" which had been provided by the League of Nations between the wars. The original convention applied only to Europe and its scope was extended to the whole world by its 1967 Protocol. Conversely its definition with time has become more restricted and it is currently seen by the UK government, not as a way of offering protection, but as a set of criteria for excluding people.

In the current UK context an asylum seeker is an individual who has applied to the UK authorities for refugee status. To apply for asylum is a legal process, (hence the term "illegal asylum seekers" sometimes seen in the press is a contradiction in terms). The Home Office uses the word refugee, not in its normal English meaning but to mean somebody who has been granted Indefinite Leave to Remain (ILR) or similar status.

Since 2006 ILR is no longer granted in the first instance. Rather you can get Discretionary Leave (DL) which is reviewed after 3 years or Humanitarian Protection (HP) which is reviewed after 5 years. Your status is then reviewed after this period; if your country is deemed to have become stable, you may be deported. ILR is only granted on review.

What is the current situation in the UK?

This is reflected in the ICAR (Information Centre for Asylum and Refugees in the UK) and UNHCR United Nations High Commissioner for Refugees) statistics.

http://www.icar.org.uk/pdf/st008.pdf

http://www.unhcr.ch/cgi-bin/texis/vtx/home?page=statistics

These statistics can be summarised as follows. The first essential is to distinguish refugees and asylum seekers from economic migrants. It is estimated that there are about 270,000 refugees and asylum seekers who have been here, in the UK, for many years (about 0.5% of the UK population) according to the United Nations High Commissioner for Refugees (UNHCR) (6). There are also 2.8 million legal economic migrants (7) and perhaps 500,000 irregular (illegal) ones (8). Economic migrants are here to work and they come because we need them for our economy. They come from the European Union, Ireland, the Indian subcontinent and other countries. To quote the Home secretary (November 2003); "there is no doubt that a large proportion of our catering and hospitality industry, particularly in London and the South-East, are relying on clandestine employment". The number of applications for asylum in Britain has fallen dramatically in recent years from 84,000 in 2002 to 18000 in 2010. The proportion of applicants granted some kind of leave, fluctuates year to year between 20% and 30%

The UK regulates economic migrants and has the right to do so. Refugees and asylum seekers are here because of our international treaty obligations, primarily the 1951 Geneva Convention and its 1967 protocol (9) but also the 1950 European Convention on Human Rights and subsequent treaties of the European Union. We have only an average number of refugees compared to other European countries, and fewer than many developing countries (10). We are tenth in frequency of asylum seekers per head of population the list of west European countries. Many poor third world countries; such as Iran, Pakistan or Tanzania, have a higher proportion of refugees than we do (11).

How does it feel to be a refugee in the UK today?(1;12;13)

The asylum seeker has to register his claim, usually at the port of entry or at Lunar House in Croydon (home of the IND immigration and nationality directorate of the home office), "as soon as possible" after arriving in the UK. If he fails to do so he is not entitled to any support. He may be detained and sent home if the immigration officer finds his application to be "clearly unfounded". Before the initial interview he may fill in an SEF (self completion) form. The home office then compares the contents of the initial substantive interview with any subsequent interviews. Differences are taken as evidence that the applicant is not genuine. Yet the original form will have been filled in by a highly traumatised person who has, almost by definition, undertaken an illegal journey whose details he feels he must hide. All asylum seekers will have been in conflict with the authorities in their home countries, perhaps 10% will have been systematically tortured. They are unlikely to reveal the full truth to the first UK government official they meet. From the home office they meet a "culture of disbelief".(1)

A substantial, but unpublished, proportion of asylum seekers are detained in specialised detention centres or in prison, often on arrival. This has much increased in recent years with "fast-track" detention. The UK is the only European country to hold asylum seekers without prescribed time limits and without judicial review. According to the institute of criminology in Cambridge, "this practice is used in an ad hoc fashion to encourage withdrawal of applications" (14). Yet asylum seekers have not been accused or convicted of any criminal activity.

While the asylum seeker is awaiting a decision from the home office his welfare is the responsibility of a branch of the home office called UKBA (UK border agency). **He or she is not allowed to work or earn money**. He will be paid restricted benefits (£36.62 for a single adult which is about 70% of equivalent income support). You could try this for yourselves, if your parents will let you. If he is willing to be dispersed out of London, he will be offered accommodation, typically in a hostel. If he chooses to stay with relatives no financial help will be given towards accommodation. Dispersal refers to the current UK policy of accommodating refugees dispersed throughout the country and not in natural areas of settlement near their relatives or community.

When an asylum seeker gets a positive decision, there is frequently an awkward transition. He is no longer the responsibility of UKBA but has the rights of an ordinary UK citizen. He has 14 days to leave UKBA accommodation and apply for ordinary social security benefits or a job and council housing, yet the paper work often takes longer than 14 days to process. During the hiatus he may be destitute and homeless. The commonest cause of destitution among asylum seekers is an administrative error at UKBA leading to a delay in payment.

The policy of dispersal means, perhaps understandably, he is offered the least desirable council accommodation in the least desirable areas of the UK. In some, areas strong anti-immigrant feeling has occurred; in others refugees have been generously welcomed. The perception on the part of both the local council and the refugee is often that if the first choice of accommodation is refused, no further accommodation need be offered.

Finally, at least two thirds of asylum seekers will see their claim eventually rejected. They become, in the terminology of the Home Office "failed asylum seekers". Some will return home, or be removed by the Home Office. Some will melt into the black economy. Some however remain here legally, if they come from countries, such as Somalia, to which the Home Office recognise that it is too dangerous to deport people. They are, however, destitute and receive nothing from the UK government. We have, in this way, created a new Dickensian underclass of people who live in our country but have no, or very restricted, rights to work, benefits, housing, or health care. They are dependent on charity or illegal work. A strong case can be made for an amnesty and some are campaigning for this (Strangers into Citizens). http://www.strangersintocitizens.org.uk/

Unaccompanied minors are a particular problem as different rules apply under 18, yet there is no objective test of a person's age. Even if they are accepted as minors, they lose many rights on reaching age 18 and may be deported back to their countries of origin.

What can refugees bring to our society?(15)

Our country has accepted many waves of refugees over the centuries. As a whole refugees tend to work hard and value education highly. Given half a chance they will contribute more to society than they have been given. The UNHCR website gives a slide show of famous refugees, including Albert Einstein, who have contributed notably to their host countries. On the UN website, and why should I not boast about her, you will find this photo of my mother who was one of the founders of the new profession of simultaneous interpretation. She worked for the UN, the OECD, and NATO, the EU and many world leaders as well as raising a family.

Reference List

(1)   Asylum voices; experiences of people seeking asylum in the United Kingdom. London: Churches Together in Britain and Ireland; 2003.

(2)   Home office research study 243 - Understanding the decision making of asylum seekers. London: Home Office; 2002.

(3)   Baker R. Psychosocial consequences for tortured refugees seeking asylum and refugee status in Europe. In: Basoglu M, editor. Torture and its consequences: current treatment approaches.Cambridge: Cambridge University Press; 1992. p. 83-106.

(4)   Silove D. The psychosocial effects of torture, mass human rights violations, and refugee trauma: Toward an integrated conceptual framework. Journal of Nervous & Mental Disease 1999;187(4):Apr-207.

(5)   Gorst-Unsworth C, Goldenberg E. Psychological Sequelae of Torture and Organised Violence Suffered by Refugees from Iraq . British Journal of Psychiatry 1998;172:90-3.

(6)   UNHCR statistics http://www.unhcr.ch/cgi-bin/texis/vtx/home?page=statistics. 2005.
Ref Type: Internet Communication

(7)   Labour migration to the UK; an IPPR fact file. London: Institute for public policy research http://www.ippr.org.uk/publicationsandreports/publication.asp?id=272 (accessed 13/09/2005); 2004.

(8)   Romero-Ortuno R. Access to health care for illegal immigrants in the EU: should we be concerned. European Journal of Health Law 2004;11:245-72.

(9)   1951 Geneva Convention and its 1967 protocol. 2005.
Ref Type: Internet Communication

(10)   ICAR. Key statistics about asylum seeker arrivals in the UK February 2005 update. 2005.
Ref Type: Internet Communication

(11)   UNHCR statistics http://www.unhcr.ch/cgi-bin/texis/vtx/home?page=statistics. 2005.
Ref Type: Internet Communication

(12)   Welcome to Britain; Voices from the front line of the refugee crisis. The Medical Foundation for the care of victims of torture; 2004.

(13)   Rutter J. Refugees: we left because we had to. 3rd ed. London: The refugee council; 2004.

(14)   Webber L, Gelsthorpe L. Deciding to detain: How decisions to detain asylum seekers are made at ports of entry. Cambridge: Institute of Criminology, University of Cambridge; 2000.

(15)   Knox K, Teichman I. Credit to the Nation: refugee contributions to the UK. London: Refugee council; 2003.

Letter to the BJGP re confidentiality of the General Practice registration process (2017)

This letter is unpublished. The editor of the BJGP, Professor Roger Jones, did suggest expanding it until I pointed out to him that the BMJ had already published a whole page article on the same subject

Dear Editor,

Recent articles in the press have made clear that the registration details of migrant patients are no longer confidential to the patient and their practice. In the last year the home office made 8,000 requests to NHS data for the registered address of specific individuals(1). Although these requests are supposed to be closely scrutinised, only 69 were rejected(2).

The legal basis is a "Memorandum of Understanding" between the Home Office and NHS data(3). Data should only be requested in adults, in those convicted of a known immigration offence, or who have failed to report as required and when all other avenues of investigation have been exhausted.

As a consequence, migrants whose paper work is not in order are likely to avoid registering with a general practice, leading to the dangers that have been listed before; it can deter vulnerable people (especially pregnant women) from getting medical help and it can lead to the spread of communicable diseases such as HIV or TB.

The context of this memorandum is that for at least a generation the Home office has been getting other government agencies to do the work of its immigration officers. First housing officers, later schools, finally hospitals and employers have been made responsible for reporting possible irregular migrants to the Home Office(4). Because GPs are not directly employed but self-employed, attempts to make general practice front-line staff fulfil the same role have so far been resisted successfully (5-8). By means of this "Memorandum of Understanding" with NHS data, the Home Office has finally succeeded in obtaining registration data (not clinical data) for irregular migrants from General Practice.

Reference List

(1)   NHS hands over patient records to Home Office for immigration crackdown. The Guardian 2017 Jan 24.

(2)   NHS patient data handed to Home Office in immigration crackdown. The Independent 2017 Jan 25.

(3)   "Memorandum of Understanding between Health and social care information centre and the Home Office and the Department of Health". 2017.
Ref Type: Statute

(4)   Cohen S. Deportation is Freedom. London: Jessica Kingsley Publishers; 2006.

(5)   Doctors should refuse to check patients' immigration status, says BMA. BMJ 2015;350(h):3468.

(6)   Vernon G, Feldman R. Government proposes to end free health care for "failed asylum seekers". BJGP 2006 Jan;56(522):59.

(7)   Vernon G. An Alarm Bell. BJGP 2008;58(549):285.

(8)   Vernon G. Denunciation; a new threat to health care for undocumented migrants. BJGP 2012;62(595):98-9.

Medicine and society

This section includes very varied pieces delivered to different audiences; their varied styles reflect the intended audience. I can only defend their inclusion on the basis that a General Practitioner should engage with is local community and play a part in its life.

The first essay is based on a portfolio item which I wrote for the MSc. It was given as a talk in the local postgraduate centre in Harlow. It was an attempt to bring some rather basic insights of sociology to the attention of practising doctors.

Professional autonomy: a good thing or a bad thing?
(unpublished)

Introduction

The question of how much professional autonomy doctors should have is a topical one. In their different ways this question has been propelled to the front page of the newspapers by Dr. Harold Shipman, Dr. Donald Irvine, and the Bristol case. It has become clear that a GP has used the cover of professional autonomy to become the biggest serial murderer in British history.

Definition

What is professional autonomy? It is a right or privilege enjoyed by doctors, it consists of independence from direct supervision by the state or patients. Like all rights it has its corresponding duties. Indeed the right cannot exist unless the other parties carry out their duties (1). Professional autonomy only exists then in so far as the other parties, patients and the state are willing to grant it. It is precisely this willingness which is changing. This autonomy extends not only to the practice of medicine but also education and even content. Autonomy of content means that the medical profession decides what is a medical problem and what is not. Autonomy of education means that doctors control the training of doctors. Doctors sometimes abuse this autonomy by using exams as a means of restricting entry to branches of the profession rather than as a means of training. This is called credentialism (2).

If a group of GPs were asked to consider what are the good and bad points of autonomy and management they might be they would come up with something like this.

	Good	Bad
autonomy	High status and pay, good for new ideas?	Alienating to patient, expensive? Dangerous?
Motivational management	should be good not just for new ideas but their implementation	may not work
bureaucratic management	homogenisation, weeds out "bad doctors"	complex, expensive, kills initiative

It would seem that while autonomy is nice for doctors it takes something away from patients in the sense of reducing their self-reliance and making them depend on doctors. This is the concept summed up in the word alienation. This implies that the patient is left less self-reliant, even if cured, by his contact with the doctor. Bureaucracy (figure 1, third row) while it can enhance equity seems to stifle life, innovation and feed-back. If it is so extreme that doctors simply do what managers tell them we can talk about the "proletarianisation" of doctors(3). The magic formula in the middle tends to be rather elusive in practice.

Autonomy from inside can be a warm and cuddly concept speaking of high status, high pay and trust. From the outside it can look quite different. In order to engage in dialogue with those who currently wish to decrease our autonomy it is first necessary to see their point of view. Below is a series of imaginary and deliberately provocative statements about dry cleaners.

Professional autonomy; the case for dry cleaners.
A1; Doctors define what health is and thereby distinguish patients' needs from patients' wants.
B1; Dry cleaners define what whiteness is thereby distinguishing what is white from what is not.
A2; the profession (with the government) sets up a NICE committee to decide what new treatments we can afford and which we cannot.
B2; Dry cleaners set up a "National institute for cleaning excellence" to decide which cleaning processes we can afford, and which shades of grey they will define as white.
A3; NICE decides there is insufficient evidence to justify the use of the anti-flu drug Relenza.
B3; Cleaners "NICE" in the absence of long-term follow-up studies of wearing slightly grey clothes on social status, ceases to support cleaning of clothes more than once a month.

Statement A1 (Doctors define what health is and thereby distinguish patients' needs from patients' wants.), sounds OK. It is what is called autonomy over the content of medicine. Statement B1 (*Dry cleaners define what whiteness is thereby distinguishing what is white from what is not.*), sounds less convincing to medical ears. We rather feel we know what is white and do not want it defined by cleaners. Clearly some of these statements are rather over the top, but I hope they show in a light-hearted way how

161

professional autonomy can look very different to someone outside the closed circle of medicine. Sociologists who have been some of our sternest critics; what have they got to say?

Sociological Theories

Sociologists have long studied the professions, including the medical profession.

Model		examples
The attribute approach	list of attributes which define a profession	Goode (1950s)
functionalist	functions performed for society	Parsons (1950s)
occupational control	position a result of power struggle	Friedson (1970s)
based on economic system	a variety	Johnson, Navarro (1970-1980)

This figure lists some well-known positions. As can be seen these positions have changed over the decades perhaps in line with society in general which has become less deferential to doctors, and in the USA sometimes frankly hostile. Goode (4) and others in the 1950s listed attributes of the professions (figure 4).

Goode's list of the attributes of a profession (adapted)
1) The profession determines its own standard of education and training.
2) The student goes through extensive socialisation.
3) Professional practise is legally recognised.
4) Licensing and admission is run by the profession.
5) Relevant legislation is shaped by the profession.
6) Practitioner relatively free of lay evaluation and control.
7) The norms of practice are more stringent than legal controls.

These are really unremarkable. From the stand-point of this essay it should be noted that items 4-7, more than half the list, arguably deal with aspects of professional autonomy. Parsons (5) at the same sort of time was describing autonomy as part of an unspoken contract with society. Doctors gained autonomy and monopoly of health care in return for using their expert knowledge and a service orientation into which they were socialised by years of training.

However far from the position of autonomy having been achieved by an unspoken contract, it was in fact the result of a power struggle in which a particular group of doctors (those who conformed to the dominant scientific paradigm of the age) (6), wrestled autonomy from the state and the public. Faced with the very powerful and unregulated American medical profession of the 1960s Friedson (7) argued as follows; either the talk of autonomy is a mere rhetoric to gain more power (as he thought it was) or autonomy (as doctors and Parsons claimed) is justified by self-regulation. He argued therefore that if doctors can be shown to fail in self-regulation then their claim to autonomy is bogus and mere rhetoric ((7) p.137).

I would suggest that this argument is false because autonomy is good in many ways (listed in figure 1), and it is not only justified by self-regulation. However, his argument is logical within its own parameters and it is important to understand that it was this argument which motivated him. Because what he actually did was to spend many months observing an American clinic in the 1960s. What he observed during that whole period was that self-regulation was limited to not referring to colleagues one did not trust and, very occasionally, a "talking-to". No other form of self-regulation actually happened in the period of observation. What he observed in the USA in the 1960s, while it no longer happens there, has been typical of my experience of British general practice (1984-2000). So he concluded that because his premise (that professional self-regulation was a sham) was confirmed, he had proven his main point (that doctors want autonomy merely as a bid for power). I am arguing however that while he did confirm his premise, this conclusion does not follow from it because professional autonomy is good in other ways than just self-regulation. This is a point I want to explore further.

GPs and the 1990 contract

Probably a good way for GPs to reflect on the good and bad sides of autonomy is to consider the imposition of the 1990 contract. It was perceived by GPs at the time as a loss of their autonomy. In that respect it made the job less attractive. Yet most GPs today would agree that some parts of the contract were better than others. Many would justify the imposition of cervical screening targets in terms of the results. At last the cervical screening program was put into order, and recently mortality from cervical cancer has even begun to drop. However, few would support the over 75 checks. There was research available at the time to show they were ineffective. Over the years they have been quietly dropped. Yet in the intervening period we were forced to pretend we were doing them and fill in forms yearly which had to be answered in a more or less "diplomatic" manner. I am suggesting that this loss of autonomy subtly corrupted our honesty and diminished the trustworthiness of our feedback to the health authority. This effect of imposing reform can be seen as part of a wider pattern. We always face the dilemma of reforming by persuasion which is slow or of reforming by force which is fast but can have perverse results. This was explained by Professor Toynbee in his history of civilisations (8). His explanation of their rise and fall was as follows. One day someone has a good idea. First he explains it to a band of disciples who follow him and all is well. Then sooner or later the disciples get impatient and impose their ideas on everybody else. Unfortunately the result of having a good idea imposed on you is not that you learn the good idea (though you may carry it out), but that you relearn the old skill of obeying orders (or often of pretending that you have obeyed them).Politically this is an accurate picture of the 1990 contract in which a few leaders of the college, tired of failing to persuade their colleagues to follow them, collaborated with the government of the day to impose their "good ideas". This was also the effect of the 1990 contract. Doctors had reinforced the pattern of learning to obey or avoid the rules rather than the pattern of learning to use their intelligence and initiative to do what is best for their patients.

The experience of the rest of the world

If we look at the history of medicine in the 20th century it seems to me we can see clearly the results of extremes of autonomy and the lack of it (figure 5).

High autonomy	Low autonomy
3rd world esp. Latin America	Totalitarian e.g. Nazi, communist
all doctors in towns, no rural health care, poor public health	some achievements in public health e.g. the Nazi anti-smoking campaign
high status for doctors	many "public health" disasters; e.g. Nazi

	euthanasia, mass famines Ukraine 1930s, China 1958
no incentive for service	no possibility of feed-back hence loss of contact with reality

In certain capitalist countries of Latin America doctors have high autonomy and status. Typically, you will find all the doctors in the capital and none in the rural areas. Public health is often poor. This was the situation in Malawi (Central Africa) where I worked. There were about 100 doctors in the country for five million people. Of these perhaps twenty worked in the rural areas where the majority of the population lived. At the other extreme are the totalitarian countries. Here autonomy of all citizens including doctors has often been reduced to near zero. There can be some benefit for public health. For example the Nazis ran an early and successful anti-smoking campaign (9), or Cuba was able to drastically reduce illiteracy. But because of lack of flexibility and feedback the most terrible things were done in some cases. For example the Nazi extermination of the mentally defective (which was led by doctors) (10), or the mass famines in the Ukraine in the 1930s or China in 1958. This last famine, engineered by man, caused many more deaths than World War II (11).

Summary

Professional autonomy then can have good and bad aspects. Autonomy cannot be justified purely on the basis of self-regulation(7) but can on the basis of enabling initiative and encouraging genuine feed-back(8). A moderate amount is probably best but it is difficult to decide how much. This is a very British view. It has however a philosophical underpinning in the work of Isaiah Berlin (12).Autonomy is of course another word for freedom. In his terms what I am saying is that freedom and equity are competing ideals. Too much freedom leads to freedom for the powerful (doctors in this case) to oppress the weak. Too much stress on equity leads to a stifling of life and often an inability to listen to feed-back. This was also the conclusion of Friedson when he looked back at his classic work twenty years later((7)p.390-392) "Without preserving a delicate balance between license and constraint, we can find ourselves enmeshed in a health care system that reduces the quality of our lives.....If doctors struggle for policies sustaining the kind of responsible and limited autonomy that is patently justified by the welfare of patients, they will find many allies to help them. "

Reference List

(1)   Weil S. L'enracinement. Paris: Gallimard, 1949.

(2)   Dove R. The diploma disease. London: Allen and Unwin, 1976.

(3)   McKinlay J, Stoeckle J. Corporatisation and the social transformation of doctoring. International Journal of Health Services 1988; 18:191-205.

(4)   Morgan M, Calnan M, Manning N. Sociological Approaches to Health and Medicine. London: Routledge, 1985.

(5)   Parsons T. The social system. New York: Free Press, 1951.

(6)   Jewson N D. The disappearance of the sick man from medical cosmology. Sociology 1976; 10:225-244.

(7)   Friedson E. Profession of medicine, with a new afterword. Chicago: The university of Chicago press, 1988.

(8)   Toynbee A. A study of history. London: Penguin, 1989.

(9) Proctor R. The anti-tobacco campaign of the Nazis; a little-known aspect of public health in Germany 1939-45. BMJ 1996; 313:1450-1453.

(10) Burleigh M. Death and Deliverance: "Euthanasia" in Germany 1900-1945. Cambridge: Cambridge University press, 1995.

(11) Vaclav Smil. China's great famine Forty years later. BMJ 1999; 319:1619-1621.

(12) Berlin I. Four essays on liberty. Oxford: Oxford paperbacks, 1989.

A Christian looks at euthanasia (2010)

This is based on a talk given at our Christian men's group in Felsted, where I live. The group was run on a Saturday morning by my friend and mentor John Dixon.

Definition

What is meant by euthanasia? The word is undoubtedly used with different meanings. Most definitions will highlight the intention, that is to say the intention to kill. The definition given by the Christian Medical Fellowship is; "Killing by action or omission of another person with or without their consent." Clearly by using the word euthanasia we imply something about the motive; that it is not theft or revenge but to end suffering. In other words, it is a particular form of killing in which the killer believes that the person being killed "has a life which is felt to be not worth living."

This sounds good as far as it goes but who is going to judge that "a life is not worth living" and how is society going to police this – there's the rub. After some further definitions I shall consider the dilemma for the individual then consider how society might respond to euthanasia.

By physician assisted suicide (PAS) we mean the situation where the physician prescribes but does not administer a medication in a dose intended to be lethal. This is clearly to be distinguished from suicide which is already legal but does not involve the doctor. In voluntary euthanasia (VE) the physician prescribes and administers the treatment with lethal intent. This is to be distinguished from treatment that eases pain or distress but may shorten life (see below.) Finally, involuntary euthanasia implies the doctor prescribes and administers the treatment with lethal intent without the consent of the patient, presumably because the patient is unconscious, is a new-born baby, or otherwise lacks capacity to decide.

Some people draw a strong line between action and omission, between giving a lethal treatment which they condemn and withholding a lifesaving action which they are inclined to condone. I will make no such strong distinction because the definition I am using emphasizes intent. As Aquinas argued many years ago acting and omitting are not so very different because by an omission we mean failing to do good, albeit not any good but only the good one ought to do.

The individual

Christians have traditionally not supported euthanasia and for a very simple reason; because the Bible tells them killing is wrong. Traditional Christians have admitted some exceptions to the ban on killing; just war and state executions. Other faiths; Islam, Judaism give their followers a similarly clear lead. For the modern agnostic decisions are altogether more difficult. However Christian thought does have some ways of thinking which can help other people.

The principle of double effect

One is the principle of double effect. This states that, although one may never do evil that good may come of it, one may carry out a good action, under certain conditions, despite the fact that one foresees a serious evil possibly resulting from it. We must, however, pay careful attention to the conditions, because, while this principle authorises some actions, it also excludes many. The four conditions are:

1. The act done must be good in itself.
2. The agent must have a right intention, that is he or she must desire the good effect and not the evil one.
3. The first effect must be good or at least equal first with the evil effect. This impedes the good effect resulting from an evil one. The good effect is not achieved by the bad effect.
4. There must be proportionately grave reason to justify the act.

Rather helpfully we can see that if the intention is to relieve pain in somebody with a serious terminal illness, it is permissible to give a pain-relieving treatment which may possibly shorten life. This principle of double effect, while helpful in some circumstances, is not without its critics and for example, has difficulty in dealing with amputations (where the good effect is achieved by means of the ill effect, amputation thus breaking principle 3 above.)

Morphine and pain

The situation with which ordinary people most often identify is the use of pain relieving drugs such as morphine in terminal care. Indeed, to read the popular press, one might think that this is what is meant by the word "euthanasia." However, the use of morphine in terminal care is not controversial in medical circles in the UK and that for two reasons. Firstly, it has been shown that, properly used, morphine does not shorten life in the terminal care setting (although large doses can kill.) Secondly, we can invoke the principle of double effect described above. Finally, pain differs from other bodily sensation in that its meaning is an integral part of its experience. I can remember a soldier who had been captured and tortured both by the enemy and by his own side. He said that the torture by his own side was more painful because it attacked not only his body, but his very self. Similarly treating pain never involves drugs alone but also an exploration of what the pain means for the patient. People who work in palliative care tell me that once the pain and anxiety have been dealt with there are often precious moments with loved ones before the end.

While certainly not saying that nobody with cancer has died in unbearable pain in recent years in the UK, in twenty-four years of general practice I do not remember a patient dying with uncontrolled pain; it is rare if appropriate resources are available.

Proportionality

Another useful concept is that of proportionality, or technically "ordinary and extra-ordinary means". What it means is that it is reasonable to require people to conserve their lives by ordinary (ordinary for their society etc.) means, but they are not obliged to conserve their lives by extra-ordinary means (e.g. second bone marrow transplant, bankrupting family etc.) In other words, a middle-aged man with a dependent family would certainly have a moral duty to accept modern treatment for a heart attack; an elderly person can legitimately accept or decline a modern cancer treatment of uncertain efficacy which may be painful or otherwise unpleasant.

The case of Alzheimer's

Alzheimer's disease poses different dilemmas. It poses in its starkest form the question; "who do we consider to be human?" For the Christian we are human because we have been created by God, and we maintain that dignity even when our mental capacities have left us. For the rationalist philosopher for whom the rights of humans are somehow linked to their intellectual capacities, there is no easy answer to the ethics of euthanasia in Alzheimer's disease.

The new mental capacity law in the UK is quite helpful in this area. A person is now judged to have capacity, not in a global way, but for each specific act. If they do not have capacity then the doctor must act in their best interest. Acting in their best interest includes finding out and taking into account the wishes of the relatives and any wishes the person themselves may have expressed when they did have capacity. In this way it is now quite legal not to pursue every medical avenue; tube feeding or hospital admission, in demented patients once these enquiries have been made.

Private moral codes and public laws – Euthanasia and the law

So far we have been considering private moral codes, but society has some interest in our moral codes. For example, while modern Britons feel suicide is a private act, most would agree that murder should be illegal, that it should be proscribed by the state. Some modern societies have allowed euthanasia. Notoriously the Nazis started with euthanasia for the mentally infirm and gradually expanded the scope of their program until Jews, Gipsies, homosexuals and others were exterminated in the Holocaust. For example, Franz Stangl, later convicted of co-responsibility for the killing of 900,000 people in the death camps of Sobibor and Treblinka, earlier in his career was commander of the killing facility at Hartheim used by the T4 euthanasia program.

Having a mother from a Jewish village in Poland where all the inhabitants (except four) were slaughtered by the Nazis during the war, this example is naturally much on my mind. Holland is the country where euthanasia is practiced most widely. It is of note that about 10% of the patients killed in this way have Alzheimer's disease. As well as voluntary euthanasia, involuntary euthanasia (of very sick premature babies and others) occurs. In Holland, unlike the UK and some European countries, the hospice movement has not taken off perhaps because people in severe pain can be offered euthanasia. Finally, in The USA state of Oregon PAS (physician assisted suicide) has been legal. The numbers here are small, but because most doctors are naturally reluctant to become involved, a small number of physicians are responsible for most of the cases that have occurred.

The slippery slope argument is the argument that once you start a euthanasia programme you do not know where it will lead. The Nazi Holocaust, where the bureaucracy and personnel involved in the euthanasia programme later became a key part of the Holocaust is the example often given. Clearly Holland and Oregon have not slipped down the slope in the same way. They do not really count as counter-examples in my eyes, because the argument is not that all stones will slide down a slippery slope, only that some may. What has happened in Oregon is the creation of a bureaucracy that sees the killing of people as something that happens to their office files, coupled with operatives whose daily work is assisting suicide. This does seem sinister to me.

In the UK polls of the public show about 55% of the public in favour of euthanasia. Polls of doctors show a substantially lower proportion and among hospice doctors the proportion is lower still (1-5 %.) There is clearly something about potentially being asked by society to do the deed that focuses the mind and turns people against euthanasia.

The possibility of improper pressure from relatives seems entirely plausible. Even without euthanasia legislation many elderly people "feel a burden" on their relatives and need reassurance on this point. Alzheimer's disease is also a burden on society and, if euthanasia were legalised, one wonders whether society would seek to treat Alzheimer's patients as well as it currently does, or fund research as generously as it currently does.

In summary I would argue strongly against the legalisation of euthanasia because of the danger it poses to society as a whole. I would rather see greater support of hospice care and better treatment of elderly demented people in our society.

References;

"The Moral Challenge of Alzheimer's disease" Stephen G Post, John Hopkins 2000

"Philosophical Medical Ethics" Raanan Gillon, Wiley 1985

"Into that darkness" Gitta Sereny, Pimlico 1974

The following talk was given to a group of men, not necessarily Christian, for a meal and a talk organised by the Anglican vicar, the Reverend Colin Taylor, on Monday evenings at a local pub.

The Health and Social Care Act 2012   (unpublished)

When our vicar asked to talk to you about the recent NHS act, I initially refused because I told him that the difference between you and me is that I know that I do not know what the outcome of the new NHS legislation will be.

(This is because the changes are permissive but not mandatory.)

I will start with a story. Many years ago, in Italy, my wife Susan and I saw a lunar eclipse. She saw the light waning as the earth threw its shadow over the moon and told me "this is a lunar eclipse." When we returned to our party, some members had seen it, others not. One however was indignant, (she was Her Majesty's British Consul in Vienna,) she said, "I have read today's Times and it was not in it, so it cannot have happened."

Human beings perceive the world through what they already know about it. Our friend knew "The Times" was reliable; this deeply influenced her perception of the world, indeed blinded her to something she could have seen with her own eyes.

This also explains how a Tory politician could say in the run up to the election that he would avoid any re-organisation of the NHS, and then propose a re-organisation which an American health economist described as "visible from outer space." In the eyes of Tory politicians, it is an unexamined assumption that markets work and state provision does not, hence change state to market provision could not, in his eyes, be a change for the worse.

The new health service act (1)

Health care will still be funded from taxation; this legislation is about increasing scope for private provision of a publicly funded service, continuing the policy of the previous government. General practice ironically is a long-standing example of the private provision of a publicly funded service, which all recent governments have sought to bring under firm central control.

If we analyse health policy in terms of the patient, the professional and the party which pays; there are two changes

1) It is now possible for CCGs (care commissioning groups) to commission care from state sector providers or private providers. In the original draft this move would have been much stronger as the regulator had to ensure that competition was upheld, meaning that the cheaper bid, usually a private one, had to be accepted. This has been watered down since. The regulator now also has to ensure the local health economy is not disrupted. In other words, this is a permissive change in how government pays the professionals; it may now be either directly or via private employing organisations.

2) The needs and wants of patients will now be represented on CCGs by GPs and "patient representatives" who will have a stronger voice than before. This is intended to change the relationship between the patient and the payer; the government in this case. It is intended to strengthen the patients' voice. However, experience to date shows the centre retaining very tight control on CCGs with little sign of increased influence for patients or indeed GPs.

3) Rather this move might be seen as not so much a delegation of power to GP's, but rather a shifting of responsibility and hence blame in a climate where resources will be shrinking and budgets tighter.

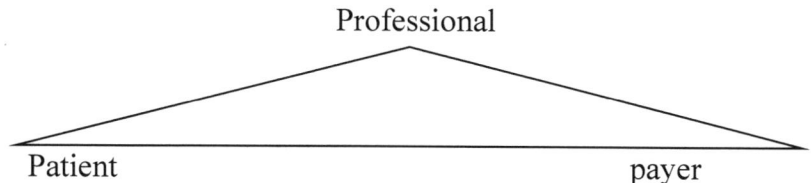

Professional

Patient   payer

The health care triangle

Historical background

The NHs was founded after WWII. Among its founding principles were clearly a desire for justice, social cohesion and a fair distribution of health resources. It was actively resisted by the medical profession, and as a result of a very British compromise, while the service continued to be funded through tax, provision was partly through private enterprise; the GPs remained private contractors.

As such a GP I am aware of some of the benefits of private provision and not ideologically opposed to it. When I started 25 years ago we did keep an eye on the opposition (the other practice in Dunmow) and this influenced us to make the practice more attractive to patients. Ironically over the last decade, while both governments have championed greater private provision (of a publicly funded service), they have regulated General Practice to such an extent that true competition occurs much less than it used to. Equally I do not believe that private provision solves all the problems of health services. We recently had a German doctor friend staying. He said that they were much further along the line of private provision in Germany, and he did not like the results. Rather I would wish to look for evidence in each instance as to which method of service delivery was most effective.

Mrs Thatcher, as is well known, reviewed the NHS. Her personal preference, I think, would have been for an insurance funded service. She was overridden by the treasury because the then NHS was so cheap. It was cheap because 80% of health service costs are staff. As a monopoly employer the NHS could keep costs down. And so the NHS was saved for a little longer.

The very simple rule is that when resources are rising and the NHS popular, the politicians like to gain the credit, and the votes. Vice versa in times of resource constraint it is necessary to find somebody else to blame.

The Blair labour government vastly increased the resources available to the NHS to bring the proportion of GNP spent in line with our European neighbours. This had some successes, particularly in cardiac services which have now reached something like the European level; before this they were woefully under-developed. Naturally the Labour government wished to retain credit for this. This meant that they put managers, as opposed to doctors, firmly in charge of the hospitals and increased their influence in primary care.

Current situation

The current situation is that the NHS budget is frozen. Compared to the cuts in other government departments this sounds generous. However, "health service inflation" runs (2 to 5%) above general inflation. This is because of the ageing population (esp. those above 85 years old), new treatments and diagnostic tests, and the decrease in social cohesion, meaning that more elderly people have to be looked after by the state.

For these reasons the health service is like the liner "Titanic" steaming towards a predictable but unseen iceberg in the path directly ahead. Realising this problem eventually almost all the professional organisations came out against the proposed changes. When savings of 20 billion are needed just to stay still is not a good time for a radical and unproven reform.

Are there any signs of this imminent crash? Can we hear the faint sounds of the iceberg beginning to scrape along the hull of the Titanic? On Saturday 14/4/2012 a record number of people attended Broomfield Casualty. As a result, ambulances were queuing up to 4 hours outside the hospital. They queue outside not because there is no room inside, but so that the hospital is not penalised for breaking the "4-hour rule." As a result, there were no ambulances to pick up sick patients. (Acting like this can occur because managers are in charge. These managers are under enormous pressure to meet targets, mainly financial targets, so that their hospitals can become "foundation trusts." One important characteristic of foundation trusts is that they can borrow money of their own right, keeping health service borrowing off the government books. The private finance initiative (PFI) is another example of the same idea; here the private sector builds a hospital and, essentially, our children pay for it.)

Michael Mandelstam has written a book; "How we treat the sick." (2) It documents the often poor standards of care in our hospitals for the elderly, especially if they are demented. It demonstrated that this is no longer a case of isolated scandals.

Since the 50s most people have been dying in hospitals. 60% of health service spend is on the last 6 weeks of life. Of course, we do not know when people are going to die. However, the current trend is to discharge people home earlier to care in the community. What this means is a visit one to four times a day by a "carer." If the elderly person has above minimum savings, they have to pay for the carer themselves. In some cases a "carer" will be funded to live with the elderly person until they die. These carers are on minimum wage. They are often immigrants. They can be wonderful people. Nevertheless, this system is growing up mainly because it is cheap; it does not take much imagination to see how it could be open to abuse.

I have talked above of social cohesion. In the health service context an example is how many elderly people are looked after by their relatives. This remains a majority but is falling. If we suppose it fell by 1% from 90% to 89%, this relatively modest fall will produce an increase in the state burden from 10% to 11%, or a 10% increase in the burden on the state. An increase of this size can be sufficient to destabilize the whole system; the "Titanic" scenario described above. The loosening of social cohesion in our societies has been demonstrated in many areas by sociologists such as Robert D. Putman, for example in his book "Bowling alone." (3)

How can we increase social cohesion?

Social cohesion is most easily increased by an external threat, real or imagined. This is how social cohesion came to be so high after WW II when the NHS was established. Bu t how can it be increased now?

This is where, in my opinion, the Christian religion has something to offer. So I will finish my talk with a story as I began it with one. I could talk about "the problem of altruism" (4) (the solution is that we often identify ourselves as a member of a group not as an individual) or the new genetics of eusocial species as in Edmund Wilson's latest book "The social conquest of the earth" (5) and I would be happy to answer questions about these, but I will finish with a story because I think you would prefer this.

"There was once a rich man who saw an exceptionally valuable diamond in a shop. Its many facets sparkled in the light. It was 3cm by 4cm making it a 20-carat diamond worth £20,000 or more. It was perfectly cut, with a pure white colour and no imperfections, which more than doubled its price. The rich man wanted it so much that he sold all he had so that he could purchase it." (Matthew 13:45-46, adapted)

Understanding God's love for us is, like this diamond for the rich man, worth more than everything we have. Because as we come to truly understand that God loves us in spite of our faults and before we have to earn his love, then we can begin to relax. As we relax into his love, we stop worrying quite so much about ourselves and have a little energy left over to care for other people. "God loved us so much that he sent his only son, Jesus, to die for us while we were still sinful." (John 3; 16-17, paraphrased.) As God is kind to us, so we can be kind to other people; that is both recognising them and treating them as "like us, of the same kind as us." Vice versa if we have to worry about ourselves all the time, we will simply not have the energy to even notice other people's needs.

In summary

The NHS is heading for the rocks. The current government's reforms are about as much use as re-arranging the deck-chairs ion the Titanic. Christians have something to offer and should be up on the bridge shouting at the captain.

Reference List

(1)   Ham C. What will the Health and Social Care Bill mean for the NHS in England? BMJ 2012 Mar 20;(344):2159.

(2)   Mandelstam M. How we treat the sick. London: Jessica Kingsley Publishers; 2011.

(3)   Putman R. Bowling alone. New York: Simon and Schuster; 2000.

(4)   Vernon G. Essay - What is man? BJGP 2003;53:504-5.

(5)   Wilson E. The social conquest of the earth. New York: Livewright publishing corporation; 2012.

Working with Polish migrants

Br J Gen Pract 2015 Mar; 65 (632): 138 -138.
http://dx.doi.org/10.3399/bjgp15X684061

Polish communities have been established in the UK for decades. After the Second World War, most of those who had fought with the allies in the Polish Army decided to stay in the UK and they formed the backbone of Polish communities for many years. With the accession of Poland to the European Union in 2004, one of the largest peacetime migrations in UK history occurred. It is estimated that 700 000 Polish migrants were in the UK in 2007, near the peak of this migration. Many have returned to Poland, but some have stayed and put down roots in this country, either as families or as single people. New Poles continue to come and go, but at a lower rate than before. In my experience, Poles are strikingly like other UK residents and just as varied, but, to run the risk of caricature, some may resemble most closely the inhabitants of a large British industrial city in the 1960s. By this I mean that smoking, drinking, and ischaemic heart disease (IHD) are highly prevalent and that mental health problems are rarely volunteered for the attention of the GP. On the other hand, most Poles will be polite to their GPs.

As EU citizens Polish people are entitled to the same health care as any other UK resident and pay the same taxes that go to fund the health service. The arcane Workers Registration Scheme (WRS), which did affect entitlement to some benefits, was abolished in 2011. Most Poles are young and fit; needing less health care than average. Many work in the care sector, especially in residential homes. Some are working in jobs below their academic qualifications. On balance, then, Poles do not present an excessive demand on the health service, but contribute substantially to it through their taxes and their work.

I am half-Polish, though not Polish-speaking, and have looked after the small number of Poles registered with our practice. In spite of the size of Polish migration the research literature is very thin.[1,2] It documents that registration with GPs by Polish immigrants was initially a problem, but seems to have improved substantially. Appointments can be a problem, especially for manual workers working long hours. Regarding health education, Poles can be a challenge. They are less likely to choose healthy behaviours than their UK counterparts and they are relatively resistant to the sort of advice available from general practice. Clearly language can be a problem. Some Poles will bring a family member or a friend as an interpreter; but many speak sufficient English if they are given time and encouragement. However, the clinical commissioning group does have a duty to provide interpreting services, either in person or telephone interpreting, when required. One specific problem in my experience is that many Poles will seek medical advice both in the UK and back in Poland. Herbal medicines are also widely used and can be bought from Polish shops in the UK. One memorable patient had an arthritis whose fluctuating severity ended up being related to the steroid injections she had received on trips back to Poland.

The names of Polish medicines can be entered on Google; their UK equivalents then become apparent. 'Google Translate' is useful for Polish words and is invaluable, for example, when working out from child health records which immunisations children have had in Poland, and which are due now. (The immunisation schedule in Poland is different from ours.) It can be used to give the Polish translation of a diagnosis, such as shingles or gout; words which few Poles are likely to know in English.

In Poland, during communist times, primary care was little developed. Primary care doctors were paid very little; less than a manual worker and had correspondingly little prestige. Even today an expectation of referral to hospital will be the norm. However, as long as the difference between the two countries is understood and explained, this need not be a source of friction. Given the high incidence of IHD, however, there should be no hesitation in appropriately referring patients with atherosclerosis. Mental health problems are even more stigmatised in Poland than they are in the UK and it is worth making it explicitly apparent to Polish patients that you are willing to talk about these issues. Overall, however, I have found looking after Poles a pleasure; the reward is well worth the slight extra challenge.

References

Burrell K (2009) *Polish migration to the UK in the 'new' European Union. After 2004* (Ashgate, Farnham).

1. Collis A, Stott N, Ross D (2010) *Workers on the move 3. European migrant workers and health in the UK: the evidence* (Keystone development Trust), http://www.keystonetrust.org.uk/documents/121.pdf(accessed 20 Jan 2015).

The NHS. Have the rivets popped?

BJGP 2017 Jul;67(660):309

When the Titanic struck an iceberg in 1912 the popular account has it that, because the ship veered to the left to avoid the iceberg, it was gashed all down its right side. As a result, water flowed into five of the separate watertight compartments and the ship sank. In fact, the Robert Ballard's submersible Argo, in 1985, found that the source of the ship's catastrophic failure was not a gash. Rather the force of the impact distorted the hull so violently that, as it buckled inwards, many of the rivets holding the steel plates of the hull popped, leading to flooding of the compartments(1).

Am I comparing the present state of the NHS to that of the Titanic shortly after it hit the iceberg? By no means. I cannot foretell the future and I do not know how long the NHS will stay afloat. Rather I wish to make a different analogy. Nobody thought the Titanic would sink; looking back, that over-confidence itself is seen to have contributed to the accident. Similarly, very few British people, be they ordinary citizens, patients, NHS employees or politicians, think that the NHS can fail and disappear rapidly. Yet complex social institutions, built up over decades can disappear rapidly; one need only open the pages of a daily newspaper to see examples of this.

A relevant example to the case of England and the NHS is the dissolution of the monasteries under Henry VIII. For centuries they had provided food, shelter and some minimum medical care to the poor and outcast of England. They depended on a social consensus that such care should be given and that monks and nuns who had dedicated their lives to this were the right people to provide it. That the monasteries would cease to exist was inconceivable. Yet, when the king decided to suppress them, the monasteries disappeared within five years (1534-1539). Two factors contributed to their sudden demise. The most pressing was the king's need for money. However, another factor was the appearance in the court of reformers who had a different understanding of the world from that of the Middle Ages and who saw charity as more of an individual than a corporate duty. The parallels to the NHS are all too clear.

It appears that some politicians have no understanding of the great dedication with which doctors and nurses, especially in their training years, look on their job, dedication without which the whole service cannot run. These politicians understand only the market model for the provision of services. This was the basis for

Lansley's 2012 Health and Social Care Act. Treating junior doctors according to this model has led to the unresolved dispute over their contract and since then to a spectacular and never previously seen loss of morale. A set of rivets gone from the structure of the NHS; gone partly because those in charge do not understand that the culture of the NHS is delicate and needs nurturing rather than wanton destruction.

The head of NHS England, Mr. Simon Stevens had asked the government for more money. Not receiving it, he has had to abandon the "eighteen week waiting list target". Abandoning this target generates savings only in the first year while the waiting lists are allowed to lengthen. Thereafter, no further savings accrue, but the waiting lists remain. Moreover, to recover the lost ground you need to spend double the money, to pay for the current patients and to catch up on the waiting list. This requires a huge cash boost such as Brown gave in the second Blair government when he was chancellor, a cash boost which is unlikely to recur. Another set of rivets gone from the structure of the NHS.

If we see the NHS as equivalent to the liner Titanic, then the iceberg, as many have pointed out, is the increasing costs of the NHS linked to an ageing population and technological progress. Will the NHS survive these changes and, if so, for how long? To repeat myself, I do not claim to be able to foretell the future. But unless we realise the speed with which a complex social institution like the NHS can be destroyed, we may, albeit unwittingly, contribute to its destruction by a foolish overconfidence that it cannot be irreversibly damaged.

References

(1) Gerald Wiessmann. Titanic and Leviathan. Darwin's Audubon.Cambrige, Ma : Perseus Publishing ; 1998. p. 269-81.

An autobiographical fragment

Bringing St Christopher back to Bobowa
(originally published in the Catholic medical quarterly 2012)

When I was a young boy I had a recurrent dream in which I took a statue of St Christopher back to Bobowa. Bobowa (Bobov in Yiddish) was the village in Poland where my mother was brought up. My mother never made any secret that her mother had been Jewish and that those inhabitants of the village who were Hassidic Jews had almost all been killed during the Second World War. A small number survived and have recreated a thriving Bobov community in New York today. I cannot remember a time when I did not know this, so she must have told us from an early age, although in those days she only rarely talked of the past.

In my first year as an undergraduate at Cambridge, reading medicine, the dream recurred once. I decided to fulfil it in a literal sense by taking a small statue of St Christopher back to Bobowa. At first my mother tried to stop me, as she had stopped my sister from visiting the year before. When she realised that I would go with or without her blessing she gave in and helped me. I went back with my sister and stayed with our aunt Ala in a small house in a wood near the village. In the village all the empty houses had been taken by local Poles. We were objects of intense curiosity as we were the first to return after the immediate post-war period. In a middle of the village, on a hillside, I found the Jewish cemetery. It was in reasonable condition which suggested to me that someone had made it their job to look after it. Aunt Ala described how during the war the Nazis had made it a "concentration village." It was surrounded by barbed wire and, on occasion, she said, she had seen the Nazis driving through it shooting the inhabitants like rabbits. Eventually all the Jews disappeared. Aunt Ala assumed that they had been taken to Auschwitz but, as I later discovered, they were taken to a forest not far away and shot (Oliner 1986).

I fell ill with diarrhoea. I was kept to my bed by this and a terrible sense of disorientation. Ala cured me with an infusion made from a local herb called in Polish "centaur's herb." The centaur is a mythical creature half man, half beast. In some sense I was coming to terms with "the beast" inside all of us human beings. Having carried my little statue of St Christopher to Bobowa I buried it there, as I remember, and thought no more of Poland for some years.

As a clinical medical student I did an elective in Magila hospital in Tanzania. While there, when the regular doctor was away for a week or two, I ran the paediatric ward. The next year I worked as a junior doctor in a London hospital. After a night on call I was woken one day by something. This time it was not a dream, since I was awake. I was woken by a presence, which I understood as an angel. I heard the message, "Go back to Africa; there is work there to do and you can do it." I cannot say that I saw an angel with the eyes of my body or heard the voice with my ears; nevertheless the presence and the message were clear. I did go back to work in Africa, though not till two and a half years later and after some hesitation on my part. My work there was very fruitful.

Some years later I entered general practice in the UK where I remained until I retired. During the early years I used to take part in the yearly spring clean at the Anglican Church. I would climb up and dust the large wooden cross on the rood screen. This was odd because I am terrified of heights and virtually blind to dust, or so my wife tells me.

It has gradually become clear to me that the dream about returning St Christopher to Bobowa had more than a literal meaning. It was something about bringing healing to hurt places. Bobowa was, as it were, the name for a deep wound in my mother's life. Working in Africa, cleaning the cross, and working in General Practice, were all outworkings of this dream which, as I see it now, shaped my life. As a child I had another dream though this one, vivid as it was, was not repeated. It was a nightmare in which I had a strong sense of vertigo, being spun round in my bedclothes while aware of a devilish Jack-in-the-box presence in the room. I was woken by a comforting presence. The vertigo ceased immediately, the Jack-in-the-box disappeared. Part of the comforting presence was the familiar sound of my father preparing his porridge for breakfast. My life has perhaps been a balance between the comforting presence of my English father and the Eastern European angst of my mother.

After many years in general practice an older GP suggested that I did an MSc in General Practice. This I did at King's and thoroughly enjoyed it. Yet at the end I was unable to get any part-time academic work, as I had hoped, in spite of trying really hard to do so, publishing papers and so on. An advert appeared for a doctor to do medico-legal work with the "Medical Foundation for the Care of Victims of Torture" (now "Freedom from torture"). This again was something which I could do and which needed to be done as working in Africa had been all those years ago. I applied and worked there one day a fortnight (more or less) for a decade.

In Essex where I live now the winter wheat is just sprouting in the fields. If you stand on the field edge looking across you can just see the odd green shoot in the brown clay soil, but no pattern emerges. If you turn your head ninety degrees and look up the furrows of the field you can see green lines of young wheat in the middle of each furrow. In the same way while you are in the middle of your active life its pattern may escape you; it is looking back that its pattern becomes clear.

References

Oliner, S. 1986. *Restless Memories; Recollections of the holocaust years.* Berkeley, California, Judah L. Magnes Museum.

Conclusion

These collected essays centre around two themes; altruism and the nature of the consultation. Altruism had seemed to me, as to many people who take the rational model of man for granted, an impossible problem, a contradiction in terms. Yet listening closely to my respondents in the qualitative study on altruism which was part of my MSc. it became clear that they did not share this model. If instead one saw man as, at least partly, socially constituted then the problem of altruism simply did not occur (I am summarising here the opening part of "Beyond altruism".) It turns out that people have different models of themselves and that understanding which model they use helps the doctor in the consultation (see; "Immunisation from compliance to concordance"). Evolutionary theory has also moved over the last decade to the view that evolutionary pressures can fall on the group or the individual, leaving us, according to the biologist Edmund O. Wilson, stuck as a species between the individual and the communal life (se; "Darwin's dream").

The other theme is the consultation in primary care. I have come increasingly to see as a form of interpretation. The doctor interprets the discourse of the patient; polyphonic(1), individual, displaying the unique "thisness" of the person, into the monophonic discourse of science which is concerned with quiddity (see; "Between thisness and quiddity"). Then the doctor interprets it back again, using the patient's language, his model of the world, which the doctor will have learnt from listening to him. Two examples of this sort of consultation are given ("Consultation after Bakhtin" and "Consultation analysis taking into account patient's view of man"). Such a form of consultation can be very powerful, the techniques not so different from those of a good salesman, so that the doctor should use it with discretion. He should remember that in past times half of what doctors thought they knew has turned out to be completely wrong. There is no reason to suppose that the same does not apply to us, only we do not know which half of what we think we know is wrong.

Am I offering a new model of the consultation? If so I would like to emphasize that the first part is more descriptive. "Thisness and quiddity" simply puts into words what happens in a consultation, any consultation in which the professional uses the quiddity (the scientific nature) of the illness rather than the thisness of the patient as a means of cure[9]. Is this description of the consultation of any use? In Molière's "Le bourgeois gentilhomme", fun is made of the hero, who is told he has been talking prose all his life and treats this as a great discovery. Is what I am saying as obvious as that? It is obvious to me now, but was not when I started on this journey. Have I used complicated words to say something simple, or found new words to express something that is only obvious once you have noticed it? The reader I am writing for, the reader every writer is writing for, is the one who, when he has read this book, says; "Yes, this is just what I wanted to say; only I had not yet quite found the words."

The second part of the model, however, is a hypothesis which could be tested, which I had hoped to test and which, maybe, a reader of this book will research. In transcribed consultations, is the patient talking in a polyphonic discourse and does the doctor respond by transposing what he has heard into the monologizing discourse of science(2)? If this is the case, it is culturally specific and can be ascribed to Western societies after 1800 according to Michel Foucault(3).

---

[9] In contrast some non-western medical systems emphasize the use of the patient's thisness and not his quiddity in treatment; in other words, they emphasize the use in his treatment of those aspects that are individual to the patient alone. Indeed, seeking out the patient's specific strengths and using them to fight his illness is an attractive concept particularly in the context of mental illness or terminal care.

Reference List

(1)   Bakhtin M. Problems in Dostoyesky's poetics. Mineapolis: University of Minesota Press; 1997.

(2)   Vernon G. The limitations of natural science as applied to medicine. BJGP 2002;52(483):870-1.

(3)   Foucault M. Naissance de la clinique- une archeologie du regard medical. Paris: Presse Universitaire de France; 1963.

ABOUT THE AUTHOR

Dr Gervase Vernon MA, MBBS, MRCP (Paeds.), FRCGP
studied medicine at Churchill College, Cambridge
and University College Hospital, London.
He also has an MSc in General Practice from King's College,
London. He has worked as a hospital doctor in Malawi,
a General Practitioner in Essex, England,
and a Medical Examiner at "Freedom from Torture" in London.
He is now retired.

Printed in Poland
by Amazon Fulfillment
Poland Sp. z o.o., Wrocław

58475381R00114